Lose Weight

Fast & For Good

A Natural Weight Loss &
Intuitive Eating Guide
For Women and Men
Who Want to Feel & Look

Great!

Julia Brianni

For permission requests or more information, connect with me

on Facebook at Julia Liss Brianni
on Instagram at julialisscoach
or email me at julia.brianni@gmail.com

I personally reply to all messages and love connecting with my readers and followers!

DISCLAIMER

The information in this book is intended for educational and entertainment purposes only. This book is not intended to be a substitute for the medical or psychological advice of a professional. Success stories and results shared do not guarantee future results or performance. Although the Author has made every effort to ensure that the information in this book was correct at press time, the Author does not assume and hereby disclaims any liability to any part for any loss, damage, or disruption directly or indirectly caused by this book. The Author and/or distributor are not responsible or legally liable for any adverse effects resulting from the use of the suggestions outlined in this book.

DEDICATION

To the people who love me, who always have my back and always make me smile, even when things don't look great. You know who you are, you fill me with infinite love and support without hesitations and I'm forever grateful to and for you.

Also, to my lovely and incredible clients all over the world who trusted me, transformed their lives for the better, and have proven that what I do is incredibly valuable, life changing, and works beautifully.

And to you—my dearest reader—for saying yes to yourself, uplifting your life, and committing to shine with your mindset and health.
You are strong, capable, and make this planet a better place.

I love you.
Thank you
for being
you.

Table of Contents

Introduction

In this book, we'll uncover all of the secrets and mysteries behind natural, permanent, and fast weight loss. You will find everything you're looking for—and more! This journey is what is going to finally allow you to experience the weight loss you desire, the beauty of deeply connecting with yourself, and also embody the amazing feeling of being at peace with what your body looks like. You know how you wish you just felt good naked? I'm warning you this might happen to you by the time you get to the end of this book! Ultimately, you will envision a new, healthy you, and you'll be able to finally love who you are. You will acquire the self-confidence you've been dreaming of in ways that are so simple and effective that you will be astonished.

We're going to be changing the way you approach food, your body, and eating altogether.

I can promise you that what I am going to share in this book has enabled me and my clients to lose extra weight <u>for good</u>— without any diets, products, or crazy exercise regimes. These methods are the exact practices that made my clients—and will make you too, when you embody them—go from feeling disconnected and ashamed when you look at yourself in the mirror to being not only happy, but actually to being *deeply in love* with your body, and maintain that over time, no matter how impossible or far away this seems to you right now.

These methods have uncovered and healed all sorts of ingrained, damaging relationships with food, and have also revealed the contorted ways and patterns we often use to interact with food. These techniques will give you the tools that you need to approach food in the most peaceful and beneficial way possible. They'll work for you regardless of circumstances. If you're enjoying a quiet meal by yourself or you're in a restaurant with a group of friends, my approach is equally effective.

The simple steps in this book will enable you to lose weight quickly and permanently, and also allow you the pleasure to deeply enjoy food—*and* your body. You can leave shame, disconnection, *and* guilt behind forever—combined with having the exact tools to face whatever is coming next in your life in the most relaxed and confident way possible.

And here is the best part:

The above can be achieved *without* dieting, restricting, *or* exercising like crazy. This means that if you're determined to lose weight without going on a food-restrictive diet, without fasting, and without cutting out your favourite foods *and* without going to the gym like it's your second home - *you can!*

The book is divided into three main parts which reflect the principles I use in my coaching practice and my proven APP method that I use with my clients:

Part one is all about <u>Awareness</u> and mindset. It's natural to want to jump straight into the practical aspects, so this is the work that most people skip, but working on your mentality, self perception and beliefs does ensure you get real results from this journey. This is probably the most life-changing work you'll ever do, you will love it -or its effect on you- and it will make everything else work like magic.

Part two is all about <u>Practice</u>. This is the action part, the work that moves the needle, that's more tangible and needs to be done. Maybe it's what you've been avoiding or that you convinced yourself it's not for you. Well, you'll be surprised how simple it really is and how it's so much easier to implement when your mindset is in the right place.

Part three is all about <u>Progress</u>. This is what helps you to make everything more pleasurable and compounds your success. It makes your improvements consistent, it makes you truly embody the new person you're becoming and reminds you how you're moving to different levels - which is exactly what you will be doing.

Let's not wait one minute longer. Let's jump right in with the methods that I have researched for years, those approaches I have experienced for myself, and which I've found benefit people <u>the most</u> with their weight loss journey—*and make sure we keep the weight off going forward!*

So, let's get ready for an incredible journey. A journey that will make you shine so *brightly,* people around you are going to be begging to know your secret!

SECTION ONE: START TO THRIVE

1.1: How To Start To Thrive In Your Weight-Loss Journey

Chapter Summary

In this chapter, you will learn:

- What the **Pole Position** is, and why it is important for your ultimate success.

- What you need exactly to thrive in your weight loss journey.

- Where your responsibility begins and ends.

- The reasons why your previous attempts have failed.

In the next chapter, you will learn what the B.P. Factor is, and how to use it to your advantage.

The Pole Position

Don't wait for the image in the mirror to change to feel connected with yourself, connect with yourself first, and then the image in the mirror will change.

Here's how:

When you want to go somewhere today, there are a lot of great resources that can take you there. This is true even if you have no idea about the way to go, or even if you—like me—have a terrible sense of orientation. If I were born even one generation ago, I would have probably spent plenty of time lost and figuring out if I needed to go right or left, even *with* a map in my hand. But, thanks to some amazing apps, it's easy now to get exactly to where I want —without wasting any time—which is awesome! I find technology mind-blowing every time I think about it. I mean, a woman named Swati Mohan just landed a rover on planet Mars.[6] Just wow!

Now, you're probably checking the cover of the book thinking, "Am I reading the right book? The one to help me get rid of my extra weight easily, while also enjoying myself? What does technology have to do with that?"

Here's what:

Technology is incredible, and its potential is huge. However, most of the time, technology is absolutely no help *unless you know what to do with it.* We, as humans, work in exactly the same way. If you wanted to go somewhere and you had your Google Map or Waze App, for instance, installed on your phone, you would open it and type in "Rome (for example)," as your destination. Where will it take you? Probably somewhere random in a huge city! This is a start, but you really have no idea where it's actually going to take you, or where you'll end up being. A similar thing happens if you only insert the street name as destination—let's say: Oxford Street—you might end up in any city in the UK, or even in the US, as there's an Oxford Street pretty much everywhere.

Only when you know exactly where you want to go, and insert the street number, the street name, the postcode, the city, the county, *and* the country, will your amazing app take you *exactly* there. How would you feel in this last scenario?

My guess is:

- You've decided your destination, which makes you excited, and looking forward to getting there. Your destination, in this instance, is how you would feel, what you would do, and what your life would look like once you've lost weight and healed your relationship with your body and with food—which is exactly what part one of this book will help you accomplish.

- You also know you're all set and have all the pieces in place to get there, the right tools and resources, like a reliable app and a charger for your phone, that makes you feel comfortable and secure —even if you don't really know all the details of the actual journey, like exactly where you'll turn right or left, or the road names you're going to travel through. Having all the pieces in place here means knowing all the key factors that contribute to natural weight loss. These are all covered in part two so you'll be equipped with all the necessary tools for a pleasurable and long-lasting weight reduction.

- So, you're doing your bit at your best, driving your car or walking, while following directions, which makes you feel more relaxed and reassured. Here, with weight loss, it means that you *commit to the journey*, even if you only take one single action every day. You have to make the conscious decision—the promise *to yourself*—that you won't give up and will trust the process, that even if the road looks unfamiliar or you feel lost (e.g., you're trying the methods in this book that may be new to you), you will keep going, *because you know it works and you are worth it.*

- You'll also be confident that you'll get to where you want to go because you'll trust that the tools will help you in the event that there's a roadblock—your app will reroute the journey for you so you don't need to worry. With sustained weight loss, confidence and faith in the journey and yourself means that *you'll trust yourself* and the process, that *you'll know that you have everything you need to get there.*

The key here is knowing where you want to go and taking action—using all the right resources. Here, you know you want to lose weight, and you've purchased this book to help you get there (well done on this, by the way!), which means you're definitely on the right track already. But let me ask you—no judgement here—has this kind of thing happened before?

What I mean by this is that perhaps this is not the first time you've decided that you wanted to lose weight? Perhaps this is not the first time you've spent your money, energy, and time to reach your goal, but, somehow, you're still dealing with this weight problem. So, it's not a thing of the past, but instead, your very current reality now?

Maybe you were very determined, and said to yourself:

"Okay, I want to lose 10 kgs, and wear a size M by June, and I'll do A and B and C to make that happen."

And then:

- That diet was too hard for you, or

- It was the wrong time for you, or

- Maybe you didn't have enough time for that fitness programme, or

- It was just too expensive, etc.

In any event, something happened that sabotaged your success, such as:

- Your accountability partner dropped out, and you couldn't find anyone else to replace them, so you also gave up on it.

- Your parent/partner/dog/cat/—insert someone important here—needed extra care from you, and you put yourself aside.

- You went on a long holiday and the food was just so good...

And so on. It all went up in smoke, and you're finding yourself right back at square one.

Well, whatever happened, let me tell you:

1. *There is nothing wrong with you.*

So, many of your behaviours might be driven by forces you have no memory of. You can't blame yourself for things you didn't even know or weren't responsible for.

For example, when my first son started attending nursery at seven months, their menu included a dessert after every meal. This meant two desserts per day for a seven-month-old baby. And they were real desserts, like chocolate fudge cake, caramel brownies - I mean real sugary, buttery stuff. Now, I'm not a dietitian or a nutritionist, but I definitely know that mind and body habits develop when you repeat the same action every day for a sustained period of time. I was totally against my son developing a sugar addiction before his very first birthday!

I was lucky enough that the nursery agreed not to give him desserts, but to give him fruit instead. However, that wasn't the case for most of the other kids. Now, I'm not saying they'll all develop a sugar addiction or become obese, but I think it's pretty clear where the chances are higher. For the sake of the story, my feedback was taken into account and shortly afterwards, all menus were completely modified and now include fruit after every meal and one dessert per week - which I find to be great!

Essentially, I'm saying there may well be parts of you that have been driving you up until now. And they were below the surface, they weren't your conscious decisions and, thus, not wholly your responsibility—up until now. We're creating a very distinct line here between the past and your present and future. And your past has no power on its own, its power over you is only the one you let it have.

Also, now that you know that so many things we do are habits, you'll be able to implement *new* habits that serve your mental and general health in great ways. This book will help you immensely with that.

2. *You were focused on the wrong things.*

For instance, the information programmed into your navigation app before starting your journey was not taking you in the right direction. An example of this is if you want to lose weight in order to be loved by an actual or prospective romantic partner. That is a very common example. Or perhaps you wanted to impress a friend. These are understandable reasons, but they're fundamentally about pleasing someone else; they're less to do with you.

When you shift from trying to please others or conforming to some external standard, and move towards responding to *yourself, trusting yourself, and embodying* your gifts, then something remarkable happens. Your whole focus shifts, and it has a massively beneficial effect on your wellbeing.

3. *The beauty of life is that you get as many chances as you give yourself.*

Are you alive? You are because you're reading this, so great! You can succeed - in your weight loss journey as well as in any other journey you desire - as long as you give yourself another chance. No matter how many times you've tried before. And I'm not saying it's all easy. I'm just saying it's possible and you're capable of succeeding. Define what success would mean specifically for *you*, not for the society you live in, not for your family or partner. Define what would make *you* feel like what you're doing and who you're being, gives you pleasure and satisfaction, and go for it.

Throughout these pages, you'll learn how to:

- Get back up from failure.

- Embrace full responsibility for your actions.

- Be kind to yourself.

- Make up your mindset so that you will be okay *no matter what*, that you will feel loved and supported *no matter what*, and that you are deeply worthy of love, *no matter what*. Because you are!

Now, in this new journey, I want you to start from the **Pole Position.** This means that you will maximise the chances of your success, and I'll be here to help you do exactly that.

You will:

- Have all the pieces in place, so that you are all set and feel safe.

- Start your journey knowing exactly where you're going—not in terms of numbers, but with regard to actual desired endpoints, so that you'll experience them much faster.

- Have all the resources that you need to get there, so that you *really* get there and you don't get lost along the way.

Putting all of the right information into your navigation app means that you automatically will start in what I call the **Pole Position**, which is the best possible starting point for you to reach the exact destination you desire.

The first section of this book is going to make sure you prepare so that you've already got a fair advantage, you've already cleared the air, and you've turbocharged your mind for success. This way, the more practical and tangible actions of section two won't be sabotaged by old behaviours or bumps along the road. Do the mindset work in this section and you'll basically guarantee your own success. I have full trust in you because I *was* you, and I know that if I can do it, you can too.

Always keep in mind that the day that matters is today, and the person you will become depends on the decisions you make today. And remember, any time you spend on you, on your mental and physical health, is *time well spent* and <u>*worth it.*</u>

→ Do you want to start in the **Pole Position**?

→ Are you ready?

→ Let's do it!

Chapter Summary

In this chapter, we looked at:

- The importance of being prepared for your journey.

- How and why previous attempts may have been unsuccessful.

- The best starting place to maximise your chances of succeeding.

1.2: A Game-Changing Factor For Your Mindset

Chapter Summary

In this chapter, you will learn:

- About the B.P. Factor, and how you can apply this concept to your life.

- A simple practice to shift even your darkest moments.

- The value of self-talk - how to use it for your advantage.

- Body dysmorphia and eating disorders.

In the next chapter, you will learn about the F.F.F work.

Your dreams are there, in your head and in your heart, for very specific reasons. I believe a sentence I once heard, which is:

"A dream doesn't come unless there's the capacity to achieve it."

I'm not sure where I heard this, but there are many, *many* inspirational quotes just like it by famous men and women throughout history. Here's some:

"Never give up on what you really want to do. A person with big dreams is more powerful than one with all the facts."

—Albert Einstein

"Dare to live the life you have dreamed for yourself. Go forward and make your dreams come true."

—Ralph Waldo Emerson

"You are never too old to set a new goal or to dream a new dream."

—C.S. Lewis

"Never abandon your dreams, you may regret it for the rest of your life."

—Fabiola Gianotti

The point is, anything is possible. If you have a rock-solid idea of exactly where you want to be in terms of your ideal relationship with your body, and of your ideal approach to food, then you'll be a lot closer to realising your goal.

To help you with getting this clear idea or vision, I'll introduce you to the B.P. goals.

Those are your **Bigger Picture** goals, which means:

- They are the final and exact destinations that you want to reach, and

- The real reasons why getting there is so important for you.

These are both essential for a great start *and* they equip you with *tons of chances to succeed.*

So, the trick here is to stop for a few minutes and truly focus your attention and imagination on the **Bigger Picture** in your life. Imagine your future—not just a snapshot, but set aside a few minutes and think about how you would *really* like it to be. But not in the ordinary way you might be used to. Here's a way that's a lot more effective, and way more fun:

    1. Don't let <u>timelines</u> be an issue. For instance, don't think it will take ages to reach the results you desire or, alternatively, that you have to rush to get there by a certain date. You're the one who controls your actions, but you're not someone who can predict the future, so open up to the endless possibilities of the universe. Have faith that things happen *for* you, *for* your benefit, *for* your highest good. The sooner you detach yourself from any time-related pressure you put on yourself, the smoother, more pleasurable, and more effective the journey becomes. And even if it took a few months to get to the point where you've lost the weight, know can keep it off effortlessly and

    2. Keep in mind that <u>the better it gets, the better it gets</u>. This is a concept I came across a few years ago and this alone majorly transformed my life and my way of being.

When you go from: *"Things can't possibly get better for me"* or *"I'm scared things will start to go wrong now that I've achieved this"* and you move towards - *"There's no other way but up, things are only getting better for me"* - that's when your entire world starts to change. And guess what, it changes for the better!

And even if unpleasant or scary things happen - like someone very close to me got Covid and I couldn't be there, and it was so painful - you know that in the grand scheme of things, everything is for you to learn, evolve, expand, and ultimately experience more awareness and joy and bring them into the world.

> 3. With regard to weight, don't consider the numbers on the scale or a specific dress size, but consider your *feelings* instead. The sooner you can get your mind to feel the feelings you're after, the sooner you'll embody them and your external circumstances will change.

For example, if you're after happiness and you focus on that feeling, you might randomly come across a joke that makes you laugh like crazy, or maybe have a conversation that makes you feel cheerful. The bottom line is that you'll already feel happy, and from that feel-happy space, you're so much more likely to take actions that create more of that quality. For example, you might well feel like you want to dance because of the happiness you're experiencing, and that will speed up your weight loss process, too. That totally makes it a win-win, right?!

Feelings are what make the difference in your life.

It's never what you have or what you don't have; it's always how you *feel* about what you have or don't have. This is why different people that have the exact same things (e.g., a lean and fit body, a pile of money, or a lack of money, and a not-so-lean body, etc.) may experience very different feelings. For instance, people with limited resources may experience happiness and fulfilment, while people who own the things we think are the ultimate possessions sometimes end up in despair, plagued by feelings of emptiness and depression.

So, the trick I want to share with you is to imagine yourself experiencing the feelings you desire to experience. I know it may be difficult at first, especially because some of those desired feelings might be the exact opposite of what you're experiencing now. I want to share my unique practice that makes this process easier and more effective.

You can get behind *feeling good*, right? So start with 'It feels good', add to it whatever else you want to experience, and the game is made. Your brain will instantly focus on the feel good part, that's like opening a door for you. Then, associate it with the rest, which is the new part that will walk through the doorway and into your mind. I use this practice regularly and it works so well every single time. I'll give some examples:

It feels good to feel light
it feels good to be free

It feels good to have plenty of energy
It feels good to be in control of what I eat
It feels good to feel connected to myself
It feels good to be an inspiration for my kids

The beauty of this is that it makes sure you feel good *now,* which is an essential part of this process. Why? Because you can not appreciate what you achieve if you can't appreciate what you already have, it's a fact. And also, I say because what's the point in waiting to feel good in a month's time when you can feel good right this moment?

And, of course, this doesn't only work within the weight loss area, it works in any area of your life. For example, are you looking for a love relationship? Then say - 'It feels good to be loved.' Or you're looking to purchase a house? 'It feels good to own my house.' You get the point, the sky's the limit!

Whatever it is you truly and deeply desire to feel, no matter how far you think this feeling is from your current reality, or even if you feel ashamed of desiring what you desire - open up, listen, and write your desires down.

Go back and read those feel-good statements again, feel them in your skin, and then add more. Think about what it would mean for you to feel these feelings. When you have an end goal in mind that's clear and wakes something up within you, you are basically giving it attention and space in your mind so it can be created and exist in your life.

Ask yourself:

→ *"What do I want the outcome to be?"*

And know:

- It's never *just* to lose some kilograms or pounds.

- It *is* what you can do with the confidence of being healthy and fit.

- It *is* how you can live your life without experiencing pain or being limited because of your weight.

- It *is* what you will think of yourself in your head when you can take care of yourself with ease and pleasure, and not worry about guilt or shame.

- It *is* what you can do with all the free time you would have if you weren't thinking about food or your body all the time.

Think about those options, and take your time to answer the following questions, always focusing on recreating the feelings you would experience if you were already there, knowing you are creating the space in your mind to make it happen in your real life:

→ How would your life be?

→ How would your relationships be?

And speaking of feelings, here's an example of how I embody this on a daily basis: I don't know the last time I checked my weight on the scale; but I observe and check in with *myself* every day, even multiple times a day, this way:

→ *"What is it that I am feeling?"*

If I like the answer, I make sure I take the time to appreciate it, and I am grateful for it. If I don't like the answer, I ask myself:

→ *"What do I want to feel instead?"*

→ *"How can I feel [a different type of feeling] instead?"*

→ *"What can I do to get there?"*

Speaking about clothes, for example, I wear any size from XS to L depending on the brand, the design, and the season, but whatever letters are on my clothes, the only thing that matters is *how I feel* and *how I want to feel.*

Do I feel or *want* to feel:

● Comfortable?

● Sexy?

● Energetic?

- Zestful?

- Vibrant?

- Positive?

- Confident?

- Self-assured?

- Attractive?

- Lively?

- Playful?

How I *want* to feel overrides any other variant. Dress sizes or numbers on the scale have no meaning for me, and they'll have no meaning for you when you decide to listen to yourself first, respond to yourself, and care about yourself - because you have a voice, and your voice matters.

Aces in the hole

It's time to talk a bit about a little practice that can help you shift those negative emotions you might be encountering. Stay with me on this because its power is incredible, and it's a free wild card that you can take out at any time.

What I am talking about is **gratitude**.

The Merriam-Webster Dictionary (the gold standard or holy grail of dictionaries) defines the word *gratitude* as a noun that means: "the state of being grateful; THANKFULNESS"[7]

Think about it. When you are thankful, you are happy for something that has already happened or that you already have. I like to think about it as diamonds, it doesn't matter how much soil there is on top, their value is incredible and when you look at them in the light they shine like nothing in this world. When you focus on being grateful, you expand your positive vibrations and shift into a different reality.

Let me give you some practical examples of how you can use gratitude any time to your advantage:

You might be thinking, "Oh, it's going to take me ages to get to a place where I feel happy with my body!" Shift this into gratitude. Think to yourself:

- *"I am so grateful I am on this journey that is taking me to a place where I feel happy with my body."*

- *"I am so grateful that I'm really doing it!"*

- *"I am so grateful that it's really happening!"*

Can you feel the power of this shift?

Let me give you another example.

If you're finding yourself in a place where you're discouraged that your old identity is trying to prevent you from moving forward, then shift this mindset into:

- *"I am so grateful about this new awareness about myself."*

- *"I am so grateful that I have decided to be kind to myself and to take care of myself."*

- *"I am so grateful that I am not alone in this, that I am loved, and that support is available and I am supported anytime I want."*

The beauty of these gratitude affirmations is that you can always add as many as you want and they will instantly shift your state, such as:

- *"I am so grateful that I have…"*

- *"I am so grateful that I am…"*

Which leads me to talk about another practice that is super effective, that is self-talk.

First of all, everybody practices some sort of self-talk. We talk to ourselves in our heads all day long, about everything. These are our thoughts and our feelings about what is happening around us. When these thoughts or feelings are directed at ourselves, we usually follow a theme, which is either positive or negative. Positive self-talk means that you talk to yourself in your head in a way that makes you feel good about yourself which means that you would be saying things to yourself like:

- *"I can totally do this."*

- *"I am doing my absolute best right now, and I'm good at it."*

- *"Yay! I'm doing it! I'm doing it!"*

- *"I am awesome at this / I'm becoming good at this."*

- *"I'm good at this, I'm excited to do it again!"*

All too often, we get stuck in a rut where we continually—whether consciously or subconsciously—criticize and put ourselves down *to ourselves!* This practice is self-defeating and causes us to sabotage our happiness, sometimes without even being aware that we are doing it.

So, take a few minutes and think about how you talk to yourself in your head. If it goes something like, "Oh, that's just great! Way to <u>screw up *again!*</u>" then you are currently practising the exact opposite of positive self-talk.

Do you think to yourself?

- *"I should be doing better."*

- *"Nothing is ever going to get better."*

- *"I look terrible/I don't like myself/I can't do this/I'm just like this."*

No one anywhere on earth gets motivated, inspired, or energized by nasty criticism. We're just not built that way, and the same goes for animals—you can look it up. Positive reinforcement in dogs is a *far* better training method than yelling, saying "NO!" a lot, hitting, or other such nonsense.[9]

What matters the most is that the *way that we talk to ourselves inside our heads* actually determines our *beliefs*, which then determine our *behaviours*. It's true. If you continually tell yourself that you are not good enough—then you won't be.

Henry Ford once said: *"If you think you can or you think you can't, either way you're right."*

If you're at the bottom of the negative self-talk pit, experts recommend doing things like saying to yourself in a mirror while standing in a wide, powerful stance (a "power pose"), with your hands on your hips, daily:

- *"I AM good enough."*

- *"I AM worthy."*

- *"I AM important."*

- *"I MATTER."*

- *"I AM smart enough."*

- *"I AM pretty/handsome enough."*

Then repeat this strategy daily until you *believe* the words that are coming out of your mouth. This is a very well-known practice. When I first started trying it, I was kind of sceptical. In fact, I was far too insecure to even look at myself in the mirror or pronounce those words so I totally understand if this feels too much for you right now. If that is the case, you can always start with affirmations that feel more authentic to you and then build up from there. For example:

- *"I AM working on myself and this is progress already."*

- *"I AM worthy of what I desire and I'm getting there."*

- *"I AM important just because I am a human being on this planet."*

- *"I MATTER to myself and I value myself and that's great - and enough."*

- *"I AM smart enough to figure this out and to keep going."*

There is a TED talk by Amy Cuddy about how our body language shapes our behaviour; it has some important information along these lines. She and some others did a study. It proved that standing in the "superman/woman" pose (with your legs spread apart and your hands on your hips) before doing something important that you're nervous about (job interview, wedding, court date, etc.) *vastly* improves your performance during the important event.[10] Now that's pretty cool!

So, if you praise yourself for your efforts and for your progress, you *will* be motivated to keep doing what you're doing, and to even *improve* on it while you're at it.

I'll give you an example from one of my past clients. She was a high-performing woman in a brilliant career with major responsibilities, and she was a mother of twins. But she didn't recognise herself anymore, didn't like her image in the mirror, and felt very disconnected from her true self. She wanted to lose weight, feel good again in her body, and stop grabbing food every time she was upset or bored. She would always start our weekly coaching sessions by saying "I could have done better." This continued until I made her notice this pattern and asked her to define what "better" would mean for her in practical terms, and also to focus on what she had actually already accomplished during the week.

This perspective shift made her alter her self-perception and behaviour. Since then, she always started with the progress she'd made, which exponentially increased from then on.

Another client of mine, a primary school teacher, decided to praise herself by giving herself stickers. She got the idea from the way she always gave stickers to her students. Every evening she found herself evaluating her day with the specific focus of finding good stuff to reward herself for. She found it fun, and it significantly increased the speed of her progress.

You can try different variations and see what works for you, but the most important thing is to shift from being your worst critic to your best supporter and ally. Shifting your self-talk from mortifying remarks to empowering and kind comments will transform you from the inside out. That means a whole new way of thinking and a whole new lifestyle. How about *that* for a change?

Always remember: you're worth it!

And if you're wondering about the science behind positive self-talk, think about this:
David Sarwer, a psychologist who is the clinical director of the Centre for Weight and Eating Disorders at the University of Pennsylvania,[32] often puts new patients in front of a mirror as a first line of frontal-attack-style treatment.

Why? The reason was simple. In order to teach his patients how to speak more kindly and gently to themselves about their bodies. The problem, he says, is that it is simply not enough for people to simply gain or lose weight. They must actually *change how they see their body in their mind's eye.*

You'd think that if you're a size small, your mind would *see* you as a size small, but that is not always the case, especially if your body image has become distorted.

Consider this: in a prominent study called, "Too Fat to Fit Through the Door," that was done in the Netherlands in 2013,[35] both anorexic women and women who did not suffer from a "disturbed body representation" walked through the same sized doors while completing a diversion task.

The women with anorexia turned their shoulders sideways to fit through, even when the doorway was *40 per cent larger* than their body size, while the other women did not.

This proved to the scientists that *how we feel* about our bodies translates into our unconscious actions, as well as how we consciously behave. These women *did not even realise* they were moving in this subtle way until they were shown a video later. Anybody could see that, in reality, their bodies were so slender that they could easily fit through the opening. But their body images were distorted. And that had a lot to do with what they'd been telling themselves in their heads for years; they believed they were far bulkier than they actually were.

Now, I'm not implying that you are anorexic at all, but there is an important parallel to draw here between how we view our bodies in our mind's eye, and what is real and true.

Do they match?

You may need to ask yourself this while standing in front of a mirror with form-fitting clothes on or with a minimal amount of clothing on. Are you seeing your body as it is? As others see it? Or are you overly critical of those curvy places, or where the clothes don't seem to fit right? Try to look at your body objectively, as if you were someone else who had never met you. How would they see you for the first time?

Now, how we perceive our bodies look in our mind's eye and how we talk to ourselves in our minds are both vital things, and we want them to be *body positive*. Dr. Branch Coslett, a cognitive neuroscientist from the University of Pennsylvania, says "...self-talk probably does shape the physiology of perception, given that other sensory perceptions—the intensity of pain, for example, or whether a certain taste is pleasing or foul, or even what we see—can be strongly influenced by opinions, assumptions, cultural biases and blind spots."

So in regular-speak, what this means is that positive self-talk is not just a transient confidence-booster. It fundamentally *changes the way we see ourselves in our mind's eye*, which, in turn, alters how we act. Speaking to ourselves in a kindly fashion, and saying encouraging words to yourself in a mirror can actually improve your body image. It can and will change your behaviour.

Let's take walking, for instance:

Confident people walk with their heads up, their backs straight, and their shoulders back. They take longer strides, and their chests are more puffed out than those of a person who is not confident, and is instead shrinking into herself. My shoulders, for example, are slightly hunched, and I believe part of the reason is this, for a long time I literally embodied my insecurities.

Take note of how you generally walk. Is it a body-positive, confident walk? What can you do about it?

In the same article (by NPR) that addressed body image and positive self-talk entitled, "Why Saying is Believing—The Science of Self-Talk," we are told that, in essence, as far as your brain goes, positive self-talk is like an *internal remodelling*.

Yes, please!

The article also points out that studies show that *how* you self-talk matters too.[36]

Here's another life-hack: When you are talking to yourself in the mirror and inside your head, try using your name instead of using the word "I".

It's a simple, but powerful tweak that could make all of the difference in how you feel about yourself. Take this quote from an interview with LeBron James, considered one of the greatest NBA players in history, when he was telling the audience how he made the decision to move to a larger market team instead of staying with the small market team that had nurtured his career from the beginning:

"One thing I didn't want to do was make an emotional decision. I wanted to do what's best for LeBron James, and to do what makes LeBron James happy."[36]

Notice how he starts out using "I" and then quickly switches to using *his own name* to describe how he made the decision that ultimately put him in the Hall of Fame. Look around. You may well notice that a lot of successful people, especially in sports where competition is so direct and intense, often describe themselves in this third-person fashion. Well, you can borrow from their example. The bottom line is that using your name when you speak to yourself is a potent way to control your thoughts, feelings, and behaviour.

So, take all of those "I" statements above, and insert your name instead of the "I" and notice how you feel about what you've said. Does it feel more real to you when you say your own name? Studies suggest that we put a lot of pressure on ourselves, and we get anxious when we use "I" statements, but that when we use our names, the anxiety and pressure goes away, and leaves a positive self-image statement instead.[36]

When I coach my clients and they open up about something they're ashamed of, maybe they felt like they fell off the wagon or they didn't meet their own expectations in certain situations, I often ask them: *if this happened to your children, best friend, [insert most beloved person for you here] what would you tell them?* I can assure you 100% of the time it's something radically different to what they were telling themselves, something so much kinder and loving and reassuring that makes them shift into empathy, understanding, hope, encouragement and clearly leaves pressure or negative judgment behind.

Going back to the feelings that you want to experience, make the conscious decision that any positive feelings you want to live in your life, you can embody them *right now*, no matter how many extra pounds you have, or how long it will take to get rid of them. This will lead you to take action accordingly, and, therefore, get to your desired result much more quickly.

Here are some wholesome and valuable decisions for you to make:

- Decide that what matters is *doing* and *being* your best *hic et nunc—here and now.*

- Decide that you acknowledge the compounding effect: many small actions, thoughts, or lifestyle changes are *not* insignificant, and that when they are multiplied and repeated, they give enormous, positive results. When you decide to believe this with your whole heart and mind, you will be well on your way to making great changes in your life—one little but effective step at a time, consistently.

- Decide that the number on the scale and the shape of your body are not the indicators of how you should feel. Decide instead that it's *you* who determines how you feel, and *your shape* will change accordingly.

- Decide that checking in with yourself and how you are feeling—*instead of* checking in with the scale on your bathroom floor—is your priority. Do this every day, multiple times per day. It's simple but so important.

If you do the above things, you will see a change in your lifestyle, your relationship with food, and your eating patterns. This is essentially why cognitive behavioural therapy is frequently more effective than antidepressant medications for depression. [37]

All that cognitive behavioural therapy really is, in a nutshell, is this—correcting distorted thoughts and exchanging them with new ones that benefit you. That's why it's so popular, and why it's effective. What it boils down to is that: Your perception is your reality. And what's the best part?

You can choose your perception.

There are many reasons why numbers on the scale or charts and statistics need to come *after* these body-positive decisions, and not before. For example, let's consider the body mass index (BMI), which you may have heard of before.

According to the National Heart, Lung, and Blood Institute, "Body mass index (BMI) is a measure of body fat based on height and weight that applies to adult men and women." Well, okay. But let's examine that statement a little further. In the past, doctors used the BMI Chart to assess a person's risk for diseases like type 2 diabetes, heart disease, some cancers, and high blood pressure. Basically, the higher the calculated number, the more at risk you are for these illnesses, based on your obesity score. According to this indicator, a person is of normal weight at a BMI of 18.5-25, overweight at 25-30, and obese if their number is over 30. However, more recent research[2] has shown that your calculated BMI is only a *rough estimate* of your body fat percentage. Like any such calculation, it tends to be less sensitive to the nuances of human individuality. It doesn't necessarily account for people who are very muscular. Such people might be on the high end of a BMI estimation, but they're not really overweight. It also doesn't take into consideration elderly people whose bodies have changed as they grew older.

In these and some other cases, the body mass index may overestimate a person's body fat percentage (e.g., athletes) or underestimate total body fat percentage (e.g., elderly people). Therefore, a BMI chart is an imperfect and unreliable tool.

Other research[2] from the Perelman School of Medicine, University of Pennsylvania, has found that the BMI chart also does not account for:

Racial differences: An Eskimo man will have a very different body fat percentage than an African woman, simply due to the differences in the climate of the regions they live in.

○ That doesn't have anything to do with them being overweight or underweight.

○ That has to do with how evolutionary changes in human beings have adapted our bodies to exist naturally in vastly different landscapes and ecosystems.

○ The Eskimo man will probably have a lot of normal, natural body fat that he needs to stay warm in an icy environment.

○ The local foods that are naturally available will also be very different from the African woman's diet. They'll be high in animal proteins and fats, instead of rich in tropical fruits and nuts.

○ We have to keep in mind that we are, after all, human animals, and that our bodies naturally adapt to our climate, even within our country if it's subject to significant variations in different areas. Let's take a geographically large nation like the USA. If we went to Florida, for instance, firstly, we would get more tanned, darker skin pretty quickly. We could well lose weight due to the high temperature and change in diet (more plant fibres and proteins, and the addition of more fish), even if we didn't exercise more.

○ The same thing happens over time to our metabolism and body fat percentage. We evolve. That's not something that we can help, it's just a fact. It's the way we are designed.

Gender differences: Women naturally and normally have a higher body fat percentage than men.

Overall body composition: It shouldn't need to be said, but people come in all types of shapes and sizes. One size (literally!) doesn't fit all, and that applies equally with BMI assessment.

Bone density: As people age, their bones become less dense as a normal part of the process.

We are all so different from one another. Sure, we are all the same species, but even identical twins have notable differences in their body type and size once they grow up (which is dependent on where they live, what they eat, and how active they are)—and they share the same DNA! That fact alone proves that we cannot look to a uniform graph or chart to tell us what we should weigh. That's just reductionist and simplistic. And, frankly, I think it's also a bit silly because I believe we're not numbers, what we are is emotional and brainy beings.

Also, some people find weighing themselves every day very beneficial and motivating, whereas, for others, it leads to obsessive and damaging behaviours like eating too much or too little compulsively which leads me to mention eating disorders.

Eating Disorders

There was a moment in my life where I could not stop obsessing over food. I would overeat all the time and constantly think about eating. I gained so much weight that I was heavier than when years later I was nine months pregnant. None of my clothes would fit anymore, and when I was with friends, I would literally put my arms on my stomach to hide the rolls, I would avoid looking at myself in the mirror, I would cringe at seeing myself in pictures because I couldn't believe that was me. And still all I wanted to do was eat. I will talk more about why I got to that point later in this book, but here I want to share a pivotal moment of that journey. One day I had just been binge eating, I don't remember exactly what it was but it was a lot, so much that I was about to feel sick. So I go to the bathroom and I catch myself thinking 'if I vomit now I won't put weight on and I can keep eating whatever I want'. In that exact moment, if I didn't know what bulimia was, I think I would have probably become bulimic. I think one of the main reasons that stopped me was that I knew what bulimia was, I recognised the pattern that was going in my mind which sounded something like binge eating and purging, and I was able to stop myself before it was too late. Knowing what bulimia was and noticing my thoughts saved me from a very common and hard eating disorder. It was hard to face the truth, but I stepped back, decided that my health and freedom came before food. Somehow I found strength and I was able to slowly but surely get better before getting worse.

This is the reason why I decided to add a few paragraphs in this book about eating disorders, so that you know what they are and you can recognise them. So you can notice your own behaviour and thoughts and act. Fast. Either to avoid getting trapped in the first place like I did, or that you can recognise that you are actually experiencing them and you can do something about it to come out sooner rather than later. And also because eating disorders and body dysmorphia may affect more people than you'd think, to the point that I would be surprised if you didn't know at least one person in your life who has or had some experience of eating disorders. As people who want to lose weight sensibly, and people who want to be kind to other people, we need to be aware of these traps along the way and be brave to confront ourselves or others around us with unfiltered, but kind and loving, eyes.

Anorexia

Anorexia nervosa is an eating disorder that is unique to developed countries. It's characterized by an intense fear of gaining weight and an individual's distorted perception of their body weight.[11] People who suffer from anorexia believe that they are "fat" or overweight when they are, in reality, usually underweight.

Symptoms of anorexia are:

- Failure to meet developmental milestones
- Thin appearance
- Exercising compulsively
- Fatigue
- Insomnia
- Thin hair
- Dehydration
- Dry skin
- Abdominal pain
- Absence of menstruation
- Intolerance to cold temperatures
- Compulsively checking out their body in a mirror
- Complaining about being overweight or fat
- Compulsively weighing themselves
- Flat mood
- Social withdrawal
- Fainting

Bulimia

Bulimia is characterised by recurrent episodes of binge eating, or eating much more than a normal person would eat. This is followed by feelings of guilt and shame, and then, most commonly, self-induced purging (vomiting) behaviour. Sometimes, bulimics will misuse diuretics, laxatives, or other medications to compensate for the food that they ate in an effort to avoid weight gain.[12] People who suffer from bulimia often feel as if they have no control over their binge eating while they are doing it. This is called compulsive behaviour. Once this has gained a hold, it can be hard to stop - but it's not impossible.

Symptoms of bulimia are:

- Rapid weight loss

- A preoccupation with weight, weight loss, caloric intake, scales, etc.

- Binge eating—eating enormous amounts of food in a short period of time

- Purging—self-induced vomiting almost immediately after eating

- Hoarding food

- Not wanting to be seen eating and not wanting to eat in public

- Drinking huge amounts of water

- Excessive exercising

- Dental erosion from stomach acid contacting teeth frequently

- Extreme concern with body weight and shape

- Mood swings

- Fainting

- Cold intolerance

- Insomnia

Body Dysmorphia

According to the Mayo Clinic, Body Dysmorphic Disorder is *"...a mental health disorder in which you can't stop thinking about one or more perceived defects or flaws in your appearance—a flaw that appears minor or can't be seen by others. But you may feel so embarrassed, ashamed, and anxious that you may avoid many social situations."*[13]

People who suffer from body dysmorphia intensely focus on their body image (sometimes looking in a mirror, studying parts of the body for hours each day) and constantly seek reassurance from others that they look okay. Their perceived "flaw" in their body causes them significant distress, takes up a lot of time, and negatively impacts their ability to function properly during daily life.

The Bottom Line

We all have some distorted thinking when it comes to our bodies, particularly those of us who are immersed (or were immersed while growing up, as most of us are) in media images of "perfect" looking bodies all of the time. In a sense, we're paying the price of this era's constant saturation in idealised standards of beauty. Whether we realise it or not, the media does have a negative impact on how we think of our bodies when we constantly see pictures and hear messages about how we should look. With the rise of social media in particular, and the advent of filters that make us look more desirable, have bigger eyes or lips, have clearer skin, etc., this problem has become worse. Unfortunately, these glossy stereotypes reinforce our negative thinking about ourselves. They can lead to a dislocated idea of what we *actually* look like. Once such thinking takes a serious hold, it can be terribly dangerous. It's important to be aware of these disorders while travelling on your weight loss journey. If you find that weight loss is becoming an obsession, or you are practising compulsive behaviours, experiencing negative symptoms—you need to seek help, simply because you are worthy of living happy and free.

And all of this underlines a significant truth that I touched on earlier. *What we tell ourselves in our heads* becomes our belief system, and our belief systems shape our behaviour. And this can be for good or ill.

It's not what's outside that matters, it's our perception of it.

This is why checking in with yourself, and your feelings—not a scale or a chart—is *imperative* when you're thinking about healthy living and your personal ideal weight.

I struggled for so long with my body not being 'enough', and was always fascinated by how people who didn't look 'perfect' but still were confident and happy with themselves. Now I can definitely say that I am in a very happy place, body and food-wise. I believe there's always room for progress, we as humans are continually evolving, but I am very satisfied with where I am, and I feel like I discovered the secrets of that confidence with my personal experience and my clients journeys too, so I'll share them with you here.

Remember - confidence and happiness does not come from your body being 'perfect.' I have visible stretch marks and loose skin, and still I happily wear a bikini, even if people notice my visibly 'imperfect' stomach. For my clients, it was their nose or their teeth, their curves, or their aging skin. I'm going to propose some ways that we can, all of us, reach a happy place and learn to be extremely happy and comfortable within our skin.

1. Focus on what you can control versus what you can't. Can I make my stretch marks disappear? No. Is being sad or upset about my stretch marks going to make them less visible or benefit me in any way? No. Am I hurting other people by not being bothered by my stretch marks? Not in the slightest. So I won't let myself be bothered by my stretch marks or any comments or looks from other people. Instead I will focus on my perception about my body and the feelings I desire to experience within my body.

2. Love your body and accept it. Perfection doesn't exist in the corporeal world, or, at best, it is extremely subjective. The only place we can find it is in our minds. Real beauty is feeling confident in your own skin.

3. Make your 8-years-old self and your 80-years-old self proud. What would your younger self be proud of? What would your older you be proud of?

Personally, I'm *grateful* for the hard times - when I couldn't bear to see my reflection in the mirror, when I refused to go on another diet, and when I decided I would find a way without wasting money on useless products. I am *grateful* because, otherwise, I wouldn't have reached the stage I'm in now. It's the place from where I've helped so many incredible people stop emotional eating, reconnect with themselves and their body, improve the quality of their health and life and love themselves and their lives. Would I have been able to understand what they were going through, been able to appreciate their damaged relationship with themselves and with food if I hadn't had exactly the same experiences myself? I doubt it very much. As it is now, I feel blessed that I can heal and help these people. My own painful experiences have enabled me to assist others to lose weight naturally and for good.

For now, I want you to know that changing and reaching your ideal situation where you are at peace and happy with your body and your eating habits *is* possible. And I can assure you it doesn't matter what your BMI is, how many times you've tried before, what your current relationship with your body is, or what your eating habits currently are. It's been done, it's real, and it's possible for you as well.

Chapter Summary

In this chapter, we considered:

- How you *feel* about yourself and the significance that can have.

- The power of positive affirmations.

- The value (or lack thereof!) of BMI assessments.

- Psychological disorders related to body image and weight reduction.

1.3: How To Find Your "Why" And Use It For Your Advantage

Chapter Summary

In this chapter, you will learn:

- The real reasons behind your journey.

- How to set intentions without feeling pressured.

In the next chapter, you will learn:

- The concept of F.F.F. work

Another key factor that gets you into the **Pole Position** is your **Why**, which is another great force and engine to take into consideration. It is a very powerful method to help you get through obstacles—and even beyond your own limits. But again, your **Why** can't be vague!

To help you be clear on that, I want you to take a few minutes to write down the answers to a few questions. You don't have to show them to anyone else; this is just for you, a way to clarify your thoughts and hopes. The simple act of taking a pen and paper is a big help in organising your aspirations. So, here we go:

→ **Why** are you on this journey?

→ **Why do you** want to be successful in your permanent weight loss?

→ **Why** is it so important for you?

If you feel that answering those particular questions is too hard, just think about it this way:

→ What would change in my life once I lost the extra weight?

→ What would change if I could eat freely without gaining weight?

→ *What if I loved my body?*

Ask yourself these questions, and don't hesitate to ask several times, until you get to the real core of it—doing this will help you so much with defining your **Bigger Picture.** There's no rush; you can put down one answer and then come back the next day with your next answer. Give yourself time and space, if need be, to reflect on the questions and the goals.

Are you doing this because:

→ Your kids are watching you, and you want to be a good example to them? Perhaps you don't want them to go through what you're going through?

→ You'd like a family and you want to increase your chances of getting pregnant?

→ You'd like to feel good in your skin while attracting a loving partner?

→ Or it might be you want to travel freely without worrying about special arrangements because of your weight?

→ Your career options could open up if you can achieve your desired weight and look?

→ Or you'll finally be able to ... [fill in the blank]?

What is your **Bigger Picture** - "**Why**"?

Focusing on the outcome and being clear on your **Why** are the key elements that will make the real difference. Always remember: Clarity on what it is that you want to achieve is directly proportionate to your chances of succeeding. I think, deep down, we all know that. Nor is it merely applicable for the goals of reaching a certain weight; it's a truism for most objectives in life.

Set up your navigation app with as many details as you can because the more details you provide, the more chances you have to get exactly where you want to get.

This is how you start from the **Pole Position**!

Action Time

Set some time aside for yourself and only yourself. Think about when it is going to be best for you, so that you will have no distractions. It can be early in the morning before you go to work, or in the evening before going to bed, or on your lunch break. Make sure that you are not distracted by anything (like your phone, your children, your pets, or other people). Yes, you might love all these things, but you pour enough emotion and energy into them during the rest of the day. Now's the time for *you*.

Finding that time—which could even be just 10 minutes—is your first step, and your game changer!

Take this "you time" to ask:

→ What are my **Bigger Picture** goals?

→ How do I *want* to feel?

→ How would my life *change* when I feel that way?

→ Why is it *so important* for me to get there?

→ Why again?

→ Why *for real?*

Really tune in with yourself, be 100% honest with yourself, and write down your answers, so that they are abundantly clear. Be kind to yourself. There's no right or wrong answer, there is just what you truly desire, which is what you're meant to experience.

It is extremely helpful to have these answers in black and white in front of you. When you've done that, you will feel and know that you're off to a great start!

Also, think about this: even a guitar played frequently needs to be tuned, so don't be afraid to do this work over and over, and come back to it—even multiple times—whenever you need clarity.

Chapter Summary

● Explore your **"Why"** and better define your **Bigger Picture** goals.

1.4: The Inner Work That Will Give You Superpowers (Because That's How You Feel When You Do It)

Chapter Summary

In this chapter, you will learn:

- About F.F.F. Work.

- About how being courageous can change both your perspective and how successful you are.

- How making solid decisions will solidify your lifestyle changes.

- How vulnerability might be uncomfortable, but helps you learn and grow.

In the next chapter, you will learn:

- That a single shift in self-perception can enhance your life enormously.

- How to switch the voice in your head so that it's constantly working for you.

- What positive affirmations are, and how their daily use helps you lose weight.

It takes a lot of courage to be who you are, but it's the most freeing and liberating experience you may ever taste. Knowing who you are, and accepting it while working to improve it, is the very first step.

Preventive measures are always better than trying to solve a problem after it's occurred. So - let's face some of the things that could have been in the way in the past so they won't get in the way again or at least you will know how to deal with them effectively.

The past has been annihilated by time and it no longer exists; that's a truth that wise people have known and taught for centuries. But you may have acquired bad habits while you were living through it - that's often the biggest problem. And they can potentially sabotage your future success. Let's deal with them right now so they don't end up becoming deal-breakers along your journey. Your past might be one of those mental blocks that is still hurting you or unconsciously holding you down.

However, I want you to know that there is absolutely nothing wrong with you if you're scared about quitting or failing. You may have done this in the past and you're worried it will happen again. Don't be - you are okay.

If you're wondering how I know this, it's because we *all* do it, myself included.

We all fall down before making it, usually multiple times. Failing, and being scared of failing, is a normal human trait. Being anxious about failure is the most ordinary feeling ever, and again—there's nothing wrong with it as long as you don't let *it* control *you*.

Let's discuss this in a little more detail.

Here are the three **F**s:

Fear is a human survival mechanism, so it's significant in and of itself. It's instinctual. But we aren't cavemen who are running around scavenging for food while avoiding a sabre-toothed tiger. We are modern-day, regular people on a weight loss/life improvement journey who want to avoid failure.

In many cases, fear is unavoidable. However, that doesn't mean it should prevent you from achieving your end goal.

Being scared doesn't mean that we can't get things done and reach our destination anyway. Being courageous essentially means *being afraid, but doing the thing we are afraid of anyway.*

The difference between being stuck in fear and achieving dreams is acknowledging the fear and doing it anyway. The alternative isn't very pretty, which is no forward motion and staying stuck and scared. That's no fun for anybody!

The winning trick here is this:

Make the **conscious decision _not_** to let your decisions be controlled by fear. Instead, acknowledge the fear, _but move anyway_. And be laser-focused on your desired outcome. You can do it!

Think about your favourite singer or, perhaps, a public figure that you admire. Think about their first concert, their first appearance on camera, or the first time they did what looks so natural for them now. I can bet they were most likely petrified with fear, but they did it all the same.

Why shouldn't you be like that? Be strong like that—scared, maybe, but _strong_. The two things are not incompatible in the least. If you make this simple decision, you can't go wrong, and there isn't any way that you _will_ go wrong because, just by being brave—you are **winning!**

Plus, _**Failing**_ and _**Risking**_ are necessary components of _**Progress**_ and _**Success**_. In fact, the more times you fail, the more chances you have to win! Looked at that way, those seemingly negative concepts - fear, risk, failing - take on a new aspect;

they're suddenly transformed into wonderful things because they're prerequisites for eventual achievement.

I'll never forget one of Michael Jordan's quotes. If you're not a sports fan, I'll let you know that he's one of the best basketball players on Earth - and he said:

"I've missed more than 9,000 shots in my career. I've lost almost 300 games. Twenty-six times, I've been trusted to take the game-winning shot, and missed. I've failed over and over and over again in my life. And that is why I succeed."[5]

The chances are even Michael's fans don't know those statistics or, if they do, they scarcely think about them. That's because there is so much success in his career it crowds out all those missed shots and lost games. Isn't that a sensational - and honest - way of looking at our supposed defeats? Failing is almost an inevitable step if you want to succeed, but keep in mind that the ultimate way of being certain to fail is to *not even try*.

Actually, that can be an insidious way our negative thoughts will trick us - "Don't try, therefore you won't fail - so that means you've sort of won." There is even a weird logic to it, but, ultimately, it's a tragic waste of our lives and potential. And, perhaps, that is the saddest kind of failure any human being can have.

So, it's okay if you've:

- Lost weight and gained it all back afterwards.

- Started a diet and didn't go all the way.

- Spent money on a gym membership that you never even used.

- Spent money on a weight loss programme and didn't follow it.

What matters is that *you're here now* with this book. Also, these things are good because failing at them means that you've learned a lot of lessons already about what you *are* and *are not* willing to do (or eat!), and you're determined to make it work no matter what. You have way more chances to win now!

So, let's go back to your **Bigger Picture** and your **Why**. There you have it, crystal clear. That's why all the previous failures don't matter, and the present and the future are what counts. This is why *success is yours*.

So, **Step One** is being okay with your **Fears**, meaning that:

- You recognise your **Fears.**

- You acknowledge your **Fears.**

- You accept your **Fears.**

- You decide to be the one in control of your **Fears.**

- You love *in spite of your* **Fears.**

Step Two is being okay with **Failure**, meaning that:

- You embrace **Failure** as a vital part of success.

- You regard **Failure** as a great chance for you to learn.

- You see **Failure** as the only way to always make progress.

Step Three is the third and last **F**, which is **Forgiveness,** and, as strange as it sounds, it's equally important as the other two **F**s, if not even more.

Forgiveness simply means:

- Making peace with yourself.

- Making peace with your past.

- Making peace with whoever and whatever is haunting you.

- Freedom

- Healing

- Power

- Peace

Being at peace—and starting fresh, and free from burdens—is not only necessary and essential for your success, but it is also crucial for the speed and quality of your progress.

Again, I want you to start in the best of all possible conditions. If you wanted to, for instance, cook a delicious meal, you would use a clean bowl, and put good, fresh ingredients in it. You wouldn't use an old, dirty bowl, would you?

This next part may feel uncomfortable, and it might even be painful. So, it might help to think about it like growing pains, for instance—like teething in babies, or like when you start exercising some new muscles you haven't used in a long time. You might want to liken it to something you did for the first time. Remember the frustration of learning to ride a bike and the number of times you overbalanced? Or driving lessons - they were even more nerve-racking! Learning to play a musical instrument was fun, but only made you realise what a lot you had to learn if you wanted to be like the guitarist in your favourite band. Or maybe you recollect trying to learn a new language?

It might feel frustrating at times, but then it eventually becomes less stuttering and awkward… and then it starts feeling good… *and then*… it becomes your new normal! Hooray!

Think about how:

- You bite into hard or chewy foods now, and you don't even remember when you were teething.

- You ride your bike now, and you love the feeling of freedom and power it gives you, but you don't think about how many times you fell in the past before riding confidently.

- You drive now and you love the comfort and convenience of your car; you get wherever you want to go without even thinking about which pedal to put your feet on.

Every one of those actions has become automatic and normal, so much so that you enjoy only the benefits now. Was it worth the initial discomfort that you hardly remember now? I'll let you answer this one, but my guess is that your answer is a resounding "*YES!*"

One trick that can help you a lot with this is taking full responsibility for yourself and your behaviour, and realising how much power and influence *you* can have over *yourself.*

You may have to do the mirror/power pose trick again, but this time, say:

"I am in control of my body and my behaviour.
I control what foods I eat and when I eat.
I am completely responsible for my own actions.
It feels good to have this power; I can become the person I want to be."

Let me tell you, I struggled with this.

For a long time, I blamed my parents and other external circumstances for my attitudes and habits. I blamed them because I was extremely insecure and my self-esteem and self-worth were low. Internally, I accused them because I had no friends, I wasn't happy with how I was and how I looked. I felt like there was no one I could be my true self with, simply because *I* was not 'enough'.

This also translated into eating issues—when I ate too much or too little, or ate food for the wrong reasons (e.g., emotional eating, or "eating your feelings"). I blamed everyone and everything *for all sorts of things* that I wasn't happy with in my life.

It turns out that I wasn't alone, and that <u>many</u> people commonly blame-shift responsibility for their life problems onto their parents. This finger-pointing at parents often continues into adulthood.I considered other people and external factors responsible for everything from my social standing to my weight, _until_ the moment I realised that ultimately:

I am my own responsibility.

It was _me_ that was the person eating too much or not eating at all. I was the one who wasn't speaking to my friends, who was isolating and being cold and insecure and never feeling enough, and therefore was completely ignored by others. I realised the one thing that would ultimately change my life for the better. No one else could change my life circumstances, the people I surrounded myself with, and when and what foods I ate. The person who could do it was _me_.

The moment that I let go of all of the accusations, anger, and resentment towards my parents—and even towards myself for blaming them—that's when _everything_ changed. I felt like I had a second chance at life!

I started thinking and acting in a different way while fully taking responsibility for my thoughts and my behaviour. I began pondering and mulling over my thoughts and actions _consciously, purposefully, intentionally, and from a much more empowered place._
It definitely was a process. It felt very uncomfortable at first, but it ultimately gave me complete and utter freedom.
Since then, I have lived every failure and every success on a _completely different level,_ and I feel like I am _living_ my life when,

before, it felt like I was in a children's board game, where I was merely a toy or pawn, a helpless plaything whose thoughts and actions were being manoeuvered by someone else.

So, to sum it up, it wasn't a five-minutes process, and it required **courage** more than anything else. The courage to confront my feelings without hiding or running away. I also had to feel that something different and better was possible for me.

The two things that helped me the most were:

- Journaling my feelings

- Talking with my coach

And I want you to know that, like everything, the more *determined* you are to achieve something, the easier you'll discover that the resources and tools you need to get there will come to you—much in the same way you've found this book.

Always remember that you're on the right path, and you're not alone.

I've said this before, and I will say it again:

- There is nothing wrong with you.

- You deserve what you desire.

- And, most importantly, you have as many chances to achieve what you want as you give yourself.

Action Time

How to Put this Plan into Practice:

- Tune in with yourself.

- Don't hide things from yourself.

- Get raw and vulnerable about your feelings.

- Write those feelings down.

- Reread and *process* the things and feelings you wrote down.

- Know that you are consciously doing this to find peace in your life.

- A pool of peace is there for you to dive in.

- Sometimes tears make it easier to slide right into the pool of peace.

- It is always okay to cry, and, in reality, crying is actually good for us.

Let's discuss crying for a minute. We've all been in a situation where we felt ashamed or embarrassed because we cried. Perhaps it was in the workplace, for instance. But, in reality, crying is how our bodies discharge stress and negative feelings. This is how we are wired. Don't believe me? According to Dr. Sideroff of UCLA, *"Crying activates the body in a healthy way...letting down one's guard and one's defences and [crying] is a very positive, healthy thing. The same thing happens when you watch a movie and it touches you and you cry... That process of opening into yourself... it's like a lock and key."*[14] In fact, in Japan, they even have *crying clubs*, called *rui katsu* (seeking tears) that meet regularly to watch tearjerker movies and cry together. Crying is good for your mental health. It releases tension and stress.[14]

The reason that crying releases tension and stress is that tears that arise from emotional distress - not the mechanical tears you get from having something in your eye - have high levels of stress hormones in them. Such tears contain an emotional regulator called manganese that helps balance your mood.

Here's another interesting quote from Dr. Sideroff: *"[Stress] tightens muscles and heightens tension, so when you cry you release some of that...[Crying] activates the parasympathetic nervous system, and restores the body to a state of balance."*[14] Crying emotional tears literally gets rid of stress. It physically expels the stress from our bodies. We may not *like* it, but it is so useful for us *to* heal and grow.

So, if you feel like you're going to cry, go ahead and do it. Feel your feelings. Crying is not a weakness, it is a strength, and it will make you feel better.

A Few More Important Questions to Ask Yourself:

1. What am I scared of? Why is *this specific thing* so scary for me?
2. What can I do to eliminate my fears?
3. What can I do to accept my fears and move forward anyway?
4. What can I learn from previous failures?
5. How do I want to deal with failure from now on?
6. Who and what do I need to **forgive** to be at peace with myself and the world?

Chapter Summary:

- The F.F.F. work is a valuable tool for success.

- Courage is necessary and good. However -

- - vulnerability is essential for growth and is also good.

- Crying releases tension and stress so can be very beneficial to you.

1.5: How To Make It All Work For You On A Daily Basis

Chapter Summary

In this chapter, you will learn:

- How powerful and empowering positive self-talk is.

- How self-perceptions shape how we behave.

- How daily affirmations can pave the way for a whole new lifestyle.

In the next chapter, you will learn:

- What the **S.W.E.E.T. M.A.P.** is, and how you can use it to your advantage.

- About what the 80/20 rule is, and how it applies to dietary changes.

- How to deal with and overcome guilt and shame and make consistent progress.

Carefully Read and Work on Internalising the Following Information

- What's going on in your *life* right now hugely depends on what's going on in your *head* right now.

- Your self-talk, your beliefs, and your ideas are the modellers that shape your reality, every day.

- It doesn't matter nearly as much what happens *around* you, but it does matter *very much* how you react to it.

- It's not the people around you, and what they're doing and saying that matters, it's what you believe about their words and actions.

- What we believe in, we act on.

How?

Because any sensory input we receive gets interpreted through our mind, our eyes, and then our paradigms and beliefs. This is not some fake science, it's a very clear fact. Our interpretations of events, experiences, and people depend on many different factors. It could be the religious traditions that surrounded us when we were growing up. Certainly, the rules or sayings our parents repeated to us when we were children have a significant impact. I can well remember my mother telling me I shouldn't step off the pavement and onto the road when cars were coming. Even now, as an adult woman (well, I like to pretend

I'm an adult sometimes!), whenever I incautiously step off the pavement, and there's traffic around, I can still hear my mother's warning.

Our education level, and what we made of it, can also be a significant influence. More generally, our beliefs about what is real and what is not and our experiences throughout life will condition our reactions.

However, the factors I've mentioned shouldn't be enough to predestine us to a certain type of lifestyle. The reason is simple - human beings are not robots; we're innately intelligent, and we can make reasoned choices.

Just to make it easy, I'll give you an example of how relative and subjective our interpretations are:

- Take, for instance, two people of different backgrounds, nationalities, traditions, and habits who fall in love. Is it impossible for them to be together and share their lives? Of course not! Yes, there may be work to do and obstacles to overcome. But understanding, compassion, empathy, compromise - and, of course, love - can make their relationship work.

- Meanwhile, siblings who've shared a great part of their lives together can be worlds apart. They may be from the same generation and have experienced the same environment and education, but they can still have fundamental disagreements. It happens many times. Blood isn't always thicker than water. Brothers and sisters may not even be able to talk to each other, so deep are the differences between them.

There are many variables in our minds. Most of what happens to us depends on how we think rather than what's happening in the outside world. And, as I mentioned earlier, there's the fact that it's always easier to blame our problems on some circumstance or person outside of ourselves, rather than looking inside and taking responsibility.

Practically speaking, if you tell yourself something like "I'm always late for appointments," you'll expect precisely that behaviour from yourself. Even worse—most of the time subconsciously—you'll make that flawed reasoning your excuse to *never* be on time. "I'm sorry I'm just like this—I'm always late—I can never be on time!" But the prophecy is self-fulfilling. You're predicting your future conduct and then carrying it out - and doing so in a negative way. This excuse, "This is just how I am," will only get you so far. Most people's common sense tells them that if you tried hard enough, were persistent, and had some forethought, you *could* change nearly any habit. This might be happening because it's happened many times in the past, or maybe because someone told you you're always late. The bottom line is that's what you *believe* and that's what you've *created* in your life.

However, if you decide to be(come) a punctual person and, even better, if you believe that you already are one—every action you take after that (both consciously and subconsciously) will reinforce your new belief. It will make you the person you want to be!

Now, considering your thoughts not only influence, but also shape your reality, think about what's going on in your mind and in your life right now.

Here are some examples—do you *believe* and keep telling yourself in your head things like this?:

- *"I'm always tired."*

- *"I have no energy."*

- *"I look terrible in every photo."*

- *"Nothing ever looks good on me."*

With these thoughts, you'll act accordingly, meaning that you'll keep doing the things that make you *even more* tired, you won't even *try* to look good in photos, and you *won't* find those clothes that flatter your figure. You're actually not looking for them! This is because:

- You expected not to find them.

- You believed you had to do the things that make you tired all of the time.

- You were convinced you always look bad in photos ("I'm not photogenic."), so why even try?

- You were sure you would look bad in any clothing, so you chose ugly, bland, loose-fitting, baggy, dumpy clothes.

Unfortunately, most negative thoughts are so frequent and so deeply ingrained they manifest in our minds, and thus into our lives, without us even realising.

There is some interesting research that shows how our brain works. The Reticular Activating System (RAS) is a bundle of nerves at our brainstem that has the important job of filtering out unnecessary information to allow the important stuff to get through. In practical terms, you know when you decide to buy a car and then suddenly you see that exact car everywhere? It's not that those cars were not there before, it's that your brain is now recording that information because you decided it's relevant. Or when you want to get pregnant and you start seeing pregnant women or babies everywhere? Or you know when you can tune out a crowd full of talking people, yet immediately snap to attention when someone says your name? Your RAS is doing its job of keeping the relevant information at the forefront and discarding the unuseful stuff. Creating a picture in your mind and giving attention to it will change your perceptions of what's out there, aka your reality. Therefore, try doing the inner work around your:

- Self-perceptions

- Fears

- Insecurities

- Judgements

- Negative self-talk

- Thoughts

- Feelings

This could be a little painful or uncomfortable, but rest assured that it will not only make you feel better straight after, but also freer, lighter, and more empowered! Doing the inner work will also get things moving and changing for you, which is a catalyst to set the ball rolling toward your new way of thinking and your new life!

The good news here is that you have the power to change things, far more so than you may have credited yourself with. With a little bit of practice, you'll master how to shift your thought patterns so that you'll *automatically* take different actions.

Guess what's going to happen after that? Your *new actions* will bring *new results* and your *new way of thinking* will show up in your life by having you experience a *new reality*. It's a much more simple process than you might think. Even if it seems very strange, it's worth trying, because it works!

Make space in your mind for your *new reality,* so that this *new reality* now has the room to exist in your life.

Action Time (1)

What are some patterns in your daily life? Reflect on these questions.

- In my **ideal situation**, how do I feel when I wake up?

- How do I feel when I look at myself in the mirror?

- What are my feelings when I'm around people?

- How do I feel when I am at work?

- In my dreams, how do I feel about these things? (A dream journal can be useful for this: keep a paper and pen by your bed and write down your dreams when you wake up. Otherwise, they'll fade away)

The "I do:" Make it Real

Well done on stretching your mind and making room for your new reality of being:

- Healthy

- Fit

- Confident

- Energetic

- Balanced

- Whatever you dream of!

So now that you've worked on your mindset, there are a few more things that you'll need to know to make your mindset shift and your new beliefs work in an effective, real, and tangible way.

The main principles to **Make it Real** are very straightforward:

→ **Decide**

→ **Commit**

→ **Believe**

→ **Persist**

→ **Repeat**

As simple as it is to write those words, it might be hard to put them into practice. This is why I want to provide you with some actionable tools to make it not only possible, but easy and pleasurable. Affirmations can help incredibly with making everything real:

- Form some affirmations.

- Write them down.

- Put them somewhere very visible (mirror, phone, post it on your desk, etc.).

- Look at them *every day.*

- Repeat them *every day,* so that they become *so much a part of you that you become one with them.*

Let's hone in on daily affirmations a little closer. A lot of people have heard about doing this, but may feel awkward trying it out. That's understandable. On the face of it, it does seem slightly odd. Standing there and talking to yourself in a mirror could even seem silly or pointless. Well, I've got some science for you that might convince you that this is a great idea!

First, your positive affirmations have to be something that specifically challenges a negative or unhelpful thought. For instance:

- Negative/unhelpful thought: "*I am not good enough.*"

- Positive affirmation: "*I AM good enough. I AM worthy. I AM loved,*" etc.

You might want to go into your Superwoman pose here. Or Superman for all you gentlemen readers. And don't be embarrassed! After all, who's watching? Only your reflection, and that's not going to tell on you.

Second, there are studies dating back to the 1980s that indicate our sense of self-integrity depends on what we say repeatedly to ourselves in our heads in positive ways.[15] More recently, positive affirmations have been proven to be effective based on "*...widely accepted and well-established psychological theory,*" according to Dr. Catherine Moore, MBA.[15] What this means is that we keep up what Dr. Moore calls a "global narrative" with ourselves in which we are:

- Moral

- Competent

- Adequate

- Flexible

- Capable of adapting to different circumstances

Now, please take notice of what Dr. Moore does *not* say we have to be telling ourselves. We don't have to try and convince our minds that we're -

- Perfect

- Exceptional

- Excellent

So, we're not exaggerating here.

Time, I think, for a small piece of artistic history. I think you'll find it interesting. In the late 1800s, Vincent Van Gogh, one of the most brilliant and talented painters of all time, and personally one of my favourites, wrote an impassioned letter to his brother, Theo, with these words:

"You don't know how paralysing it is, that stare from a blank canvas that says to the painter, 'You can't do anything.' […] Many painters are afraid of the blank canvas, but the blank canvas is afraid of the truly passionate painter who dares, and who has once broken the spell of 'You can't.'"[16]

Even a genius like Van Gogh experienced self-doubt. But that didn't stop him.

The bottom line is that: *We Are Enough*, and *We Can*, whenever we allow ourselves.
So, repeat after me: **"I Am Enough."**

Well done! Honestly, if you're here, it means you're above average—many people never get past chapter one of a book or skip the mindset work altogether. That speaks volumes about you getting to the finish line like a winner!

Everybody's "enough" is different. You have to decide what *you truly value* in your life that is *part of your identity*—"*I am intelligent.*" "*I am a hard worker.*" "*I am a good person.*" "*I'm willing to work on myself and improve*"—and focus on building that up.

It is inflexible, rigid, black and white thinking that gets us in trouble. Blame and rigid thinking have been studied, and are well known to be damaging to our mental health. The inability to change your mind is the inability—or refusal—to see a situation from a different perspective. That's always damaging because it creates barriers and it completely cuts out room for growth, progress, and improvement. Blame can make us feel heavy, like we're carrying the weight of the world on our shoulders, and can be very toxic in the long run by making forward motion and/or personal growth impossible.

Blame and rigid thinking together can make us think about things continuously and obsessively, for instance, that: "*I'm terrible because I am so fat, and I have to lose weight at all costs.*"

In this specific case, blame and rigid thinking, when combined, are the birthplace of eating disorders; they are a way that we punish ourselves mentally, and we think and think about one specific idea over and over, while reinforcing negative emotions directed at ourselves. This is counterproductive and serves no purpose except to make the problem worse. It also makes them seem much, much larger than they actually are. This is distorted thinking, and it can be very easy to fall into the trap. Still, it is just as easy to shift into a different kind of thinking that serves you once you recognise what's going on. If you become aware of your negative thinking, acknowledge it, accept it as something of the past, and forgive yourself, then good things will happen. You can then focus all your attention on opening up to new possibilities and a far better life than you've experienced. .

Very important note here: you don't have to do this work alone. The only thing you have to do alone is make the decision about the direction you want to take and what your desired outcome is—you can go back to chapter one and answer the prompts again and again to get clarity on that. The next sections will help you immensely too. Plenty of help is available to guide you, keep you accountable, and get you there. I personally coach clients 1on1 and in groups and many other great coaches and professionals are out there too, with the great purpose to be there for you, make your journey easier and effective, and see you win!

The bottom line is :

We are all imperfect people. And that is definitely okay and very normal. Own your imperfections, forgive yourself, while you work on your next level like it's the most normal and smartest thing to do. Always appreciate what you have and be grateful, while you happily work to reach new heights. Support is available and gets you to what you want faster and with more ease and pleasure, you are worthy so don't hesitate to ask.

Everything starts with your decision making.

- Deciding makes you step into your power.

- Deciding makes you take full responsibility.

- Deciding is like turning on the keys so that the engine starts.

So, here are some daily affirmations to begin with:

- *"I decide to make this health and happiness journey a priority for me."*

- *"I decide that this is bigger than dieting, exercising, and quick fixes and I'm ready for it."*

- *"I decide that I'm enthusiastic about this journey because it's going to change my life for the better."*

- *"I decide that it's going to be easy and fun."*

- *"I decide that I'll make the most of every day."*

- *"I decide that this is my life, uplifted!"*

How do daily affirmations work? Positive affirmations are a way that we can overcome negative self-talk. They're also a proven method by which we can challenge self-sabotaging behaviours. For instance, research has shown that spending just a few minutes thinking about your best qualities can help you perform better at work, and in high-pressure situations such as an interview or a meeting with your boss.[42] These simple steps can calm your nerves and increase your confidence in a meaningful way, especially in a situation that would usually induce anxiety.

So, how does this translate into our dietary habits? Daily affirmations are powerful statements that help us stick to our commitments, build our confidence, and increase our self-worth. This technique is now routinely used to treat many mental health disorders; this includes problems such as depression and low self-esteem. Studies show that a strong sense of self-worth makes it much more likely that you'll make positive changes to improve your own well-being.[43] What this means, in a practical sense, is that if you're concerned that you eat too much and don't exercise sufficiently, then going through a quick list of your good qualities every day will make it far more likely that you'll make permanent behaviour changes that benefit your health.

NEXT:

These daily affirmations need to be followed up with a rock-solid commitment.

Being committed means:

- The things that I have decided are not negotiable.

- My goals are a priority.

- These decisions need to be respected fully.

- I am dedicated to the things that I decided. They matter in my everyday life more than other things that are relatively unimportant.

You can say:

- I commit to take great care of myself *every day*.

- I commit to consider my health and wellness *my priority*.

- I commit to being positive, enjoying the journey, and appreciating myself and my life *every day*.

- I commit to being kind to myself and learning from my mistakes *every time*.

Strengthening these beliefs will shape your new reality and help you step into the feelings that you want to experience. Affirmations make you stronger and more confident. For more affirmations that will help you change your beliefs, repeat after me:

- I believe I deserve to be healthy and happy.

- I believe I can reach my goals 100 percent.

- I believe that I am not alone.

- I believe that I'm always supported by the Universe / God / Source.

- I believe that I am on my way to my best self.

- I believe that I am worthy of being happy, energetic, and confident.

Persistence and perseverance will help you overcome obstacles and keep you going when life starts throwing difficulties at you. These valuable, long-lasting characteristics will also help you when you simply get tired or impatient!

Keep telling yourself the truth:

- As long as I do my bits every day, I will see and experience positive results.

- It doesn't matter exactly *when* I get to my goal; the important thing is that it is already happening *right now*.

- No matter what others' judgments are, I'm doing this for me and this is enough.

- I want to become a better person, and -

- I can do it, I am worthy!

Here's a little Life Hack from me to you:

I have a little corkboard in my home office on which I wrote my favourite mantras and affirmations. I have affirmations on my google calendar that come up on my phone at certain times every day, I have a vision board on my desktop, I have a Pinterest vision board too. It's like making my brain—consciously and subconsciously—focus all of the time on what I want to achieve. It makes me effortlessly dive into my desired reality and it feels so good to imagine myself in there, knowing what I desire is on its way to me. Try it, it really works!

Remember that you can do more than you think you can. You're stronger than you think you are, more loved than you may think. And you deserve more than you've come to expect.

Clearing up your inner words and thoughts, owning your power, and making space for your new you is going to be an entire lifestyle change. Deciding that you're going to become the person you want to be, with ease and fun, is the very foundation of your super successful journey. So, if you haven't done it already, it's time for you to get started and get this mindset work going!

Action Time (2)

Make your own lists of:

- Decisions

- Commitments

- Beliefs

- Persistence affirmations

Then, make them ultra-visible, so that you're reminded of them on a daily basis!

Fun fact: The beauty of this method is that it works for whatever area you apply it. Whether it be your health, your relationships, or your career, you can count on it to have effect.

Chapter Summary:

- Positive self-talk is incredibly important.

- Positive daily affirmations help change your behaviour.

- Rock-solid decisions are what will make it permanent.

- You are enough!

SECTION TWO:
THE S.W.E.E.T. M.A.P.

Chapter Summary

In this chapter, you will learn:

- How small lifestyle changes can and will make an enormous difference in your life.
- What the 80/20 rule is, and how it can apply to your lifestyle and dietary changes.
- The importance of repetition and the importance of keeping an open mind.
- What the **S.W.E.E.T. M.A.P.** is, and how to use it to your advantage.

In the next chapter, you will learn:

- About the Positive Spiral.
- What *Nullus Die Sine Linea* Means, and How to Use it To Your Advantage.
- How to exponentially increase your self confidence almost instantly

At this point, it's super-important to appreciate how *daily actions* are what will shape not only your body, but your life.

These are small tweaks to your daily routine that, when added all together, equal a significant lifestyle change. I want to reinforce the idea here that there's no magic pill or mysterious secret. The whole process is so much simpler than you can imagine. It's completely achievable. I can tell you that 99% of my clients got back to me and said they were surprised that following a few simple steps could lead to such major changes in their weight, overall mood, confidence level, and, fundamentally, their entire life. And that all happened because they really committed to the mindset work we talked about in Chapter One.

However, I don't want to fully spoil the endgame's awesome surprise for you, so let's start with your **S.W.E.E.T. M.A.P.** to easy, sustainable weight loss. Let's get started!

Four essential things to keep in mind while reading this chapter are as follows:

1. It's the small things that make a difference.

It's true. Small lifestyle changes always add up to big results. Science is on my side here. Take, for example, a study done on older (average age 72 years old) women in which researchers wanted to know if the number of steps a woman takes per day has any impact on her lifespan.[38] The answer is yes!

Senior women who took an average of 4,400 steps per day, compared with women who took an average of 2,700 steps per day, had lower mortality rates after four years from *all causes.* Now, this was a study that involved nearly 17,000 women, so the researchers really did their, uh, legwork, if you will, on this one. So, even increasing your activity levels by a *small margin* has a *big impact* on your health.

Other health studies have shown the same kinds of results. In another study done on adults aged between 58 and 99, researchers found that adding just one cup of dark, leafy greens to these people's diets per day increased and protected the participants' memories and recall abilities significantly.[39]

The salad-eating people had the memory of a person *11 years younger* (!!) than they actually were, and they were studied for a span of almost five years. Now that's just incredible! Another thing about dark, leafy greens is that they're packed with Vitamin K, which many people are deficient in. Vitamin K helps a lot with exercise, stamina, and mobility, especially as we age.[40] You can get more than 100 per cent of your daily value of this ingredient by just adding one cup of spinach or kale to your meals.

If you don't love the taste of spinach or kale, try blending a handful of it into your morning smoothie—you won't even taste it! Also, you can add dark, leafy greens to your scrambled eggs or pasta sauce if you're looking to avoid their flavour or texture.

2. We need to be reminded more often than we need to be instructed.

In this section, you might find yourself coming across something that you've heard before, and that's ok because truth be told, most of us instinctively know the right things to do to improve our lives, and control our weight. We just need to be reminded and sometimes approach things from a different angle and repeat them long enough to get the results we're looking for. If you have any doubts about the importance of reminders, let me enlighten you. First of all, we know that a habit is something that we do as a matter of routine. Bad habits are a problem, but consider this: whether it's a good or bad habit you're engaged in, *it's a habit*, and it's entrenched in your mind as something you do without thinking too much about it. The solution to *bad habits* is to replace them with *good habits*. What we need to do is to get from creating reminders to building habits. Anything that you do repeatedly for long enough will become your default position. Different people have different learning curves, so some people pick up new habits faster than others. Either way, the point is to keep doing what's good for you, what makes you feel good and what's truly beneficial for you on a deep level. This is important when it comes to your relationship with food and what you do and don't eat regularly. The same goes for how active you are every day.

So, how do we get a behaviour to become routine? Triggers and reminders! And how do we trigger a reminder? It's simple. I like to ask myself *"what would make it nearly impossible that I don't get to do it?"* For example, if you want to remember to bring something to work with you tomorrow, you might put that something by the front door so that you can't possibly forget it. This is your trigger to tell yourself you wanted to take it to work. We have to do simple things that interrupt our daily life in order to remember our new habits. This is the same deal with kitchen timers and alarm clocks—when they ring, we know what to do next—pull dinner out of the oven or wake up for the day.

Nearly all phones now come with a calendar schedule and associated alarms built right into them. Use this to your advantage. You are usually somewhere within hearing distance of your phone, right? Set reminders in your phone's calendar schedule if you need to remember to do something that you don't normally do. And set it for every day.

Put a reminder in your phone and post it notes on the door to walk the dog—or, if you don't have a dog, just to take a walk—every day at 7pm, no matter what. You'll be doing yourself (and your dog) a favour, and, after a month or so, it will become something you don't even have to think about. Or put a reminder in your phone to drink a glass of water or maybe something specific that does good for your mind and body - 7am every day, recurring ones so you can't forget about them!

3. Approach everything with an open mind.

Ask yourself, "How can this apply to me?" This is the best way to learn, the only way to make it personal, and the most effective method of making it lasting and sustainable. Being open to what's possible, being open to learn, being open to try new things instead of judging them in advance is a huge skill that anyone of us can develop. It's like opening doors and finding marvels instead of keeping them shut because we think we already know what's inside.

4. The 80/20 Rule

Another extremely important concept that has literally changed my life and that I apply every single day is the **80/20 rule**. The **80/20 rule**, also known as the Pareto principle, the principle of factor sparsity, or the law of the vital few - this rule has been around since 1896, so it's been renamed a lot. It's based on the principle that approximately 80 percent of all consequences come from 20 percent of all causes in any given situation.

Italian economist Vilfredo Pareto[16] came up with this rule after he noticed the pattern in wealth distribution. He was the first one to point out that 80 per cent of the land in Italy was owned at that time by about 20 percent of the population. He did surveys of other countries, and was surprised to find the same distribution of wealth.

This power law, as it's called, translates into nature, physics, business, and even dieting and lifestyle changes. For example, in business, managers often note that 80 per cent of sales come from 20 percent of the total clients.

In the United States, for instance, 80-90% of taxes are paid by the top 20 per cent of earners in the country. Microsoft applied this law in 2002, and noted that when they fixed their top 20 percent of most-reported user problems and errors, the other 80 percent of crashes and related errors in any given system fixed themselves. These are just a couple of examples.

How this translates into dietary changes is this—if you stick to eating healthy, high protein foods with whole grains, healthy fats, and lots of fruit and vegetables 80 percent of the time, you can give yourself the leeway to snack on sugary foods or have a dessert or soft drink the other 20 per cent of the time and when you do, you can skip the usual guilty feelings altogether!

When you follow the **80/20 rule** every day, you'll never again feel obligated to say, "Oh, I can't eat that. I'm on a diet." You might say instead, "I can have a piece of chocolate cake today because I've been eating super healthy meals all week". This is a much more permissive and realistic approach than a strict diet regime. The ethos of such spartan plans is based on restrictions. They often feel like a punishment, something to tolerate until you can stop when you've reached your weight-loss goal. And we all know that as humans, our instinct is to want what we don't have- we have curly hair and want straight hair? For women, maybe you have big breasts and want smaller ones or vice versa? For men, maybe you have slender arms and you want huge, rippling biceps? Sounds familiar? Another example is when you are told not to think about chocolate, for example, or snow. Your brain will go there straight away and do exactly what it is told not to do! The solution here is to trick our mind. We win when we adopt the view that we can always have everything, but simply choose to have or not have something. That, ultimately, is the truth of the matter. And, if we do that, our brain won't push us to what we can't have.

So many of my clients came to me frustrated that they managed to stick to a diet for enough time to lose weight, but when the diet stopped they gained the weight back with interest. That is because a diet or a restrictive regime is not sustainable over a long period of time. Diets as such do not teach your mind or your body how to keep the weight off. What you need for permanent weight loss is something different, something sustainable.

What I'm talking about is an entire lifestyle change that is easily sustainable and means that you'll never have to diet again.

Chapter Summary

- Bad habits, and how to alter them into good ones. You do this through -

- Small consistent actions, and reminders, both mental and practical.

- An open mind opens doors

- The Pareto principle, and how it applies to diet.

2.1 S: Sleep - How To Leverage Good Sleep For Weight Loss

Chapter Summary

In this chapter, you will learn:

- The value of proper sleep.

- Ways to improve your sleeping patterns.

In the next chapter, you will learn:

- The value of water in your diet.

Let's start with the most undervalued thing in most of our lives: **Sleep.** This might seem a straightforward subject. Sleep is easy - we just do it. And if we stay up late a few nights, surely there's no harm done? Well, read on; lack of sleep can be subtly damaging, and it's the kind of problem that easily slips under our radar.

Sleep is an essential function because it, "*...allows your body and mind to recharge, leaving you refreshed and alert when you wake up.*"[17] Sleep allows our bodies to repair any damage done to them during the previous day, as well as to stave off infections or diseases that might be lurking in our bodies.

Without a good night's sleep, we suffer serious consequences to our ability to concentrate, our memory, and our ability to process information. We become unable to make reasonable decisions or to think clearly at all.

According to the Centers for Disease Control and Prevention (CDC), being sleep-deprived has much the same consequences as drunk-driving. Researchers found that:

○ Being awake for 18 hours has the same driving consequences as having a blood alcohol level (BAC) of 0.05%.[18]

○ Being awake for 24 hours is the equivalent of having a BAC of 0.10%, which is over the legal limit in the United States.

○ Even if you don't actually fall asleep while driving, "drowsy driving" affects your ability to focus, make good decisions, and significantly slows your reaction time.[18]

○ Drowsiness compounds the effects of any alcohol consumption, even low amounts, which makes a driving accident much more likely.[19-20]

I'd been sleep-deprived for nearly a year when my first son was born. Trust me, I know what it feels like. My brain was fried. I would forget the car keys in the car and leave the car parked with the keys inside, I would stop in the middle of a sentence because the words wouldn't come up. It was probably the most challenging time of my life. When it was over and I got back to sleeping enough hours, I felt like a new person. This is no figure of speech or exaggeration. You know how you feel when you come out of the water after holding your breath for a long time and finally feel your lungs filling up with fresh air? That's how I felt. And that's why I've never underestimated the effects of sleep on my daily life since then.

The following are some excellent "Good Sleep Life Hacks," and may be a game changer for you if you suffer from poor-quality sleep. Good sleep has been scientifically proven to help you exercise more, eat less, and be healthier overall, so let's find out some great ways to get that good night's sleep that you've been dreaming of![21]

- A reduction of blue light exposure before bed (no screens for one or two hours before bed). Try taking a bath instead, reading a book, or spending quality time with your partner or just yourself.

- A reduction of daytime napping. It tends to adversely affect your proper sleep pattern. You can still relax without sleeping!

- Supplementing with melatonin.

- A reduction of alcohol consumption at night.

- Setting your bedroom temperature for 18°C or below.

- Taking a before-bed shower or bath.

- Treatment for any sleep disorders you might have.

- Avoiding eating or drinking anything late at night to prevent sleep disruptions.

- Getting enough exercise—but not right before bed.

- Getting a weighted blanket.

- Avoiding caffeine late in the day.

- Increasing bright light exposure during the day.[21]

You don't need all of those in place. Just experiment, be curious, and observe yourself. To give you an example, what works for me is wearing an eye mask for complete darkness, keeping the room temperature low and well ventilated (heating in my bedroom is always off and I keep the windows open most of the time), and a weighted blanket. Also, this might seem like a given, but having a comfortable mattress, pillow, and bed can make all the difference in the world as far as your sleep quality goes.

Now you may ask: how can I know the quality of my sleep? Firstly, there's many tracking systems like watches or rings that track sleep and tell you all about your different phases of light and deep sleep. It is not random that they're becoming more and more popular, the importance of good sleep is huge for mental and physical good health and more and more people are realising this. Also, when you have a good sleep, you will feel like your body is very heavy and becomes lighter while waking up, and remembering your dreams is also an indicator that you've slept deeply. Or, simplest of all, you just feel incredibly good and in a very happy and relaxed mood when you wake up for no apparent reason!

Chapter Summary

We've just looked at:

- Scientific studies showing the perils of sleep-deprivation.

- Simple methods to get great and soothing night's rest.

2.2 W - Water: What To Do With It In A New and Exciting Way

Chapter Summary

In this chapter, you will learn:

- The powerful benefits of water.
- How to increase water intake easily and simply.
- The dangers of fizzy drinks.

In the next chapter, you will learn:

- Why and how to avoid excessive negative discipline in your diet.
- The value of frequent but small meals.

Time for a quick fairy story! A wizard shows up at your cottage door. He tells you he has a magic potion that can....

- Accelerate your weight loss.

- Make your skin look smoother and younger.

- Increase your physical performance and stamina.

- Boost your brain function and energy significantly.

- Reduce and even cure headaches, and -

- Relieve constipation.[22] (This is a very gritty fairy story I'm describing)

Would you drink this magic potion? Take the quill pen and sign on the parchment contract immediately? Of course you would! Well, there's no need to travel to a mythical land to get this elixir. The good news is that it's easily available here, and it's called **water**!

Water is going to be your new best friend on your weight loss/loving yourself/lifestyle changes journey!

We are made of around 60 percent water[22] and our body needs it to thrive and survive. Our brain needs it, too. Probably you already know about some of the benefits of drinking more water, but I'll mention my favourite ones below to refresh your memory. Then, we'll dive straight into what you can do to make sure you experience all the benefits yourself. We want to get some action going here, *but* we also want to make sure that it's easy, fun, and pleasurable. That way, we feel happy doing it. The routine lasts and doesn't seem like a chore.

Similarly to a fish tank, if you change the water manually once a month, it will take you longer to remove the dirt and make it nice and clean. It's a much more messy business than if you cleaned it once a week. Also, maybe some of the dirt will still stay there even after cleaning because it's too stuck on.

However, if you have an automatic system that injects fresh, clean water and takes the old water away every day, you won't need to worry about cleaning the tank manually at all.

In the past, I researched and tried many different face creams because I was obsessed with my skin, and I was dismayed it looked so dry; it made me look much older than I was. But then a great beautician, who also happens to be a friend of mine, told me: "What is the point of trying to cure the outside, if you don't heal the inside?"

Increasing my water intake has completely changed my skin! It's so much smoother now, so much softer, and nowhere *near* as dry as it was before. So, if you want healthier and better-looking skin, use the cheapest *but most effective anti-age product available* - water! I still use face creams, but the results are much better and more visible now than before because I'm helping from the inside out.

According to the School of Medicine and Public Health at the University of Wisconsin, drinking at least eight glasses of water per day will make your skin more radiant and help rid the body and skin of toxins.[23]

When you feel like you have no energy and you're getting headaches or even back pain, your body is highly likely to be dehydrated. Water really helps keep every cell lubricated and keeps the muscles elastic. As a result, you are less likely to experience discomfort.

A simple, easy, free, huge help from the inside that makes a big difference in the quality of your living is drinking enough water. And, naturally, when you feel good and have no aches and pains, you perform better.

But how does it help with weight loss? It takes up space in your stomach, so its volume makes you feel fuller and reduces hunger automatically. It makes you eat less, which helps digestion and prevents constipation. Hello, nearly effortless weight loss!

It's a fact that when you increase your water intake, you'll experience a general increase in your well-being. However, there's one small drawback that you might not enjoy—you'll start going to the toilet a lot more. You'll be like a pregnant woman who constantly needs to pee! This may be annoying at the beginning, but I want you to think about it this way:

Your body is getting rid of toxins and cleaning your system, so it's a sort of catharsis, or a full body purification, where you release the bad and come out lighter and cleaner. I know this sounds dramatic for a simple wee! But that's the way I love to look at it, as I believe—and you've probably figured it out by now—that a positive mindset is everything.

And here's the *Dulcis in fundo*, or icing on the cake—I once listened to an interview of a guy named Rich Menga,[25] who is a musician, among other things, who went from owning nothing to building an empire. When he was asked: "What's the secret to your success?" He replied: *'As crazy as it sounds, my secret is <u>drinking three litres of water a day.</u>"*

Let me tell you something about *my* life experience with water. The difference water makes to how sharp, fresh, active, positive, and productive my brain is now has honestly amazed me. It almost (but not quite!) leaves me speechless because it's such a huge improvement. I've experienced it myself *and* have gotten the same feedback from all my clients; now I never, ever work without a pint or a bottle of water next to my laptop!

Also, as a bonus, let me mention here how much money you'll save and how much sugar you will be sparing your body when you drink water instead of juices, flavoured drinks, or soda.

So, do you want to:

- Have tons more energy?

- Feel healthy within your body and mind?

- Sharpen and freshen your brain?

- Have better-looking, glowing skin?

- Lose weight effortlessly?

Of course, you do! And water helps with *ALL* of that!

On the other hand, perhaps you're thinking...

- *"I don't like water."*

- *"I'm never thirsty."*

- *"I always forget about water."*

- *"Water is so bland and boring."*

Well, don't worry, because I've got you covered. Here are a list of things you can do to make drinking water easy and pleasurable:

- Add a slice of lemon/orange/lime/grapefruit/a slice of ginger.

- Add some natural herbs that you like, for example, broken mint leaves.

- Drink herbal teas—hot or cold; there are great ones that don't have any caffeine, and which taste delicious. They make it easier to drink more.

- Type 'drink water' or 'water reminder' in your app store/google store and download an app to remind you to drink and also to keep track of the amount you drink every day. You can have hourly reminders on your phone for this.

- Keep a bottle handy. It can be on your desk, next to your bed, in your car, and in your handbag. Make sure you've got it right there next to you all the time.

Write down how much water you consume in a daily journal—or even a digital sticky note on your laptop—and also the changes you notice in your skin, energy, mind, and mood. I'll make a good bet that you're going to notice enough positive changes to decide to stop buying sugary drinks.

I'm not a doctor, and I don't want to beat you over the head with consequential, negative information, but I *do* want to tell you exactly how much sugar is in most soft drinks.

- If you Google right now (as of March, 2021) how much sugar there is in one can of average soda (12 fluid ounces), it will tell you: ***39 grams***.[25]

- That's the equivalent of more than ***eight sugar cubes.***

- Furthermore, get this: in one 20oz (the standard size) drink, you will have consumed *65 grams of sugar, which is equal to 240 calories.* And that's not even food.

- No wonder many people think of soda drinks as "liquid candy."

- So, you can indulge once in a while, but not every day, and certainly not multiple times per day.

- Your body and teeth will thank you, I promise.

While we're about it, if you are consuming high amounts of sugar on a daily basis, you're going to have a tough time losing weight, so let's talk a bit about the benefits of cutting sugar out of your diet:

- Boost in energy level.

- Decreased body-wide inflammation.

- Increased ability to concentrate.

- Fewer headaches.

- Fewer hormonal imbalances.

- Fewer mood swings.

- Reduced risk of many diseases, some of which can be debilitating or even fatal.

Another thing is that the other ingredients in soda are bad for you, too. We've known for years that daily soda drinking is linked to obesity, diabetes, kidney damage, and certain cancers, but more recent findings have even linked soda to an increased risk of heart attack and stroke.[27]

Further, in a 2017 study, researchers found that soda consumption increased both the risks of strokes *and* Alzheimer's disease.[28]

Basically, soda is a mixture of sugar thrown in with a lot of chemicals, and the whole drink is then carbonated. Yes, it tastes good, but it can ruin your teeth, body, and even your life. This chemical soup might satisfy a sugar craving, but so would a piece of fresh fruit, without all of the risks and other garbage that your body doesn't need—and has to work hard to filter out. Also, natural sugars contain vitamins and minerals that aren't present in refined, bleached, and processed sugars.

Okay, I'm thirsty just because I've had to write this, so have you grabbed your water yet? Even if it's just a sip now and a sip later—every little helps!

This brings me on to another simple topic. **Sitting** for prolonged periods of time can be bad for your health. Another perk of drinking more water is that you are forced to move more. Let's discuss sitting a bit. Did you know that there is now a debate among health experts, with some calling sitting "the new smoking"? Take this quote, for instance, from an article that the Mayo Clinic put out in 2020:

"They [(the health risks of sitting)] include obesity and a cluster of conditions—increased blood pressure, high blood sugar, excess body fat around the waist and abnormal cholesterol levels—that make up metabolic syndrome. Too much sitting overall and prolonged

periods of sitting also seem to increase the risk of death from cardiovascular disease and cancer. Any extended sitting—such as at a desk, behind a wheel or in front of a screen—can be harmful. An analysis of 13 studies of sitting time and activity levels found that those who sat for more than eight hours a day with no physical activity had a risk of dying similar to the risks of dying posed by obesity and smoking." [24]

That is quite a shocking analysis. But the problem can be averted. Easy, small changes to your lifestyle that can mean less sitting are:

- Getting up from your office desk every hour to take a lap around the office and stretch.

- Pausing a movie or TV show to get up from the sofa, walk around, and get a drink of water at least every hour.

- Taking the stairs instead of the elevator to get to places like the toilet in public places.

These things count, and overall, you'll move your body a lot more just by doing them.

So think of drinking more water in a positive light, as in:

You're doing something powerful for your wellbeing *and* weight loss all via a simple and natural action.

Next, we'll talk about the first **E** in the **S.W.E.E.T. M.A.P.**

Chapter Summary

- We've looked at the benefits of water for your skin, brain, and body.

- Soda drinks have little that's good about them - replace them with water or other healthy alternatives, at least 80% of the time!

- Cut down on your sitting time by taking regular breaks.

2.3.1 E - Eating: How To Eat the Foods You Love And Still Lose Weight

Chapter Summary

In this chapter, you will learn:

- Why we're not going to pursue stringent diet plans.

- How effective small, frequent meals can be.

- A suggested meal schedule through the day, including snacks.

In the next chapter, you will learn about:

- The problem of emotional eating and how to effectively deal with it.

"I never thought that I would be able to eat 'freely' without gaining weight."
This is what a client of mine shared with me after starting to follow my techniques. So let's start with rule number one, which is to:

Avoid extremes

This means no hard and fast rules about cutting things out of your diet completely, and no major restrictions that are unreasonable or unrealistic. Why? Simply because none of that is sustainable. Yes, you might lose some weight if you adopt these methods, but ultimately it's too much of a burden to carry for most people. It's highly likely you'll slip, and start to get all that weight back with interest. So, we're not going to go down the road of demanding that you:

- Have no more sugar whatsoever.

- Avoid all fat.

- Ban desserts.

- Must skip meals.

- Engage in fasting.

Always remember to keep in mind the **80/20 rule**, and get enough **Sleep** and **Water**, and let's focus on the eating now.

The number one trick that works really well is ***eating more often, but in smaller portions.***

Eating small portions more often during the day will help your metabolism, so that your body can absorb and get rid of what it needs with much less effort. That's because your body has—

and knows it has—a frequent turnover. When your body is reassured that food will be coming in regularly, it won't store extra stuff. It won't hold on to excess for fear that it won't get any more.

Eating smaller meals frequently will also regulate your hunger, so that it becomes predictable and manageable. That's great if you want to feel more in control. It becomes important here to keep a sort of regularity.

For example, you can put alarms on your phone when it's time to have your meals, and it's super important to start to listen to your body. Personally, when I feel *truly* hungry, I feel discomfort in my stomach, and I start to feel that I have low energy and I am more irritable. Some develop headaches, and sometimes have problems focusing. I emphasised the word 'truly' there. That's so we understand the difference between genuine hunger and wanting food for other reasons—we'll talk about this later in the emotional eating chapter.

Soon, your body will be telling you that it's lunchtime, or that it's time to eat some nutritious food, and it will provide you with a sense of calmness and energy throughout the day.

The best option is to have about five meals per day, with three main meals—breakfast, lunch, dinner—and two or three snacks, which could be something like:

- Fresh fruit.

- A few baby carrots, or other fresh vegetables like cucumber.

- Oats.

- Dried edamame.

- Greek yoghurt.

- Roasted lupini or broad beans.

- Pumpkin seeds.

- Roasted chickpeas.

- Dried fruit.

- Almonds, cashews, pistachios, or other nuts.

- A piece of dark chocolate.

The reason that eating smaller meals makes your metabolism work more efficiently is that when you skip meals or fast, your body responds as if you are starving, or there is no food available. It slows the metabolism way down, simply to keep you alive. When you eat smaller, frequent meals, your body functions better because it has access to constant fuel, which also keeps your blood sugar levels stabilised. When your body has a more efficient metabolism, it is more efficient at using carbohydrates, fat, and protein as fuel.

I'm going to quickly mention type II diabetes here, and how most people don't seem to realise that it can happen to anybody. Even people without a family history of diabetes can develop it over time if they consume too much sugar on a regular basis and/or become obese. But I'm not going to write here all the bad things that can happen, it would be a bit like the image of damaged lungs on a cigarette package. For the smoker who wants to smoke and doesn't care about quitting, that disturbing image won't have any effect. But you're different. You want to change your eating habits—not because you don't want to get diabetes (well, maybe that too), but because you want to finally feel free, really feel good about your body, and increase your self-confidence and connection with yourself. This will give you so much more time and joy back, and more opportunities to do what you desire in your day-to-day life.

Moreover, the treatment for diabetes usually involves massive dietary shifts, especially in the way a person consumes foods and sugars (as well as supplementing the body with additional insulin), so why not change your diet now, so that you can still eat all the food you want? Act proactively, instead of waiting until you have no choice and you have to cut out a whole range of foods and drinks altogether. You're smart, you are perfectly capable, and again, you are worth it.

Chapter Summary

- We've looked at the shortcomings of the more rigorous diets.

- We've considered the value of smaller but more frequent meals, how they place less pressure on your body and your mental discipline, and help with your metabolism.

2.3.2 : Emotional Eating and Craving

Chapter Summary

In this chapter, you will learn:

- How emotional eating is stimulated.

- Four potential situations in which you may be caught up in eating for emotional gratification.

- A number of ways you can overcome these problems.

In the next chapter, you will learn about:

- Food addictions and how to deal with them.

"I discovered in a very short time the reason why my diets have failed so often in the past and what was holding me back. Now I'm 10lbs down but, most importantly, I'm mentally stronger, happier, and able to recognise when I'm at my worst. Instead of going to dive into comfort food, I do something else, and it's not even an active decision any more; it's my new normal."

This is what another client of mine shared after just a few weeks of working together.

Most of us are familiar with emotional eating. We know that when we are stressed out, eating makes us feel better. It happens because there's a reward circuit in the brain, involving dopamine. It's stimulated when we eat high-fat or high-sugar foods.

The most obvious problem with emotional eating is that it doesn't solve the underlying issue. If you're stressed because a colleague is giving you a hard time at work, you go home and eat junk food. That distracts you and makes you feel better in the moment, but doesn't rectify the problem with the colleague in any way, so you're likely to find yourself in the exact same spot the next day. If we understand what the cause of stress is and what we can do to solve it—for example in this case having a one-on-one meeting with our colleague and trying to improve the relationship—then we eliminate the cause of emotional eating.

So, how to stop emotional eating?

Well, it has to do with recognizing the triggers, interrupting the habit, and then replacing it with a stress-reliever that is actually good for us. Keeping a food diary that includes not only what you ate, but how you felt at the time you were eating it, can help. Find out *when* you experience those cravings so that it's easier to identify which one is your reason behind it. Here's a list of possible situations; all you need to do during a week is listen to your body and understand which one of those situations you relate to the most.

You crave a specific or any food:

A. When you are alone, maybe straight after meeting a specific person or after specific experiences with a person (e.g., being intimate with your partner, going for lunch with a friend) or when you are in a specific place, e.g. only at or after work, only at home, only when with someone, or straight after being with one particular person.

B. During specific times of the day, e.g., during the morning or late at night, or in the middle of the night.

C. When you feel intense emotions, like you're extremely happy, sad, or stressed out, when some particular event happens and you feel overwhelmed, or experience strong feelings and emotions.

D. None of the above, *and* it's always a specific type of food.

Start observing and studying yourself, listen to your body and keep track of that for a few days and then see if you find a recurring pattern. Make sure you write things down, either on your phone or in a notebook, so that you can keep track of this pattern once you identify it. Or use the trackers provided in this book in chapter 2.5

Have a look here at the related reasons for each category and the ways to deal with each of them. Feel free to focus on one in particular if you've discovered a pattern. You can also try more than one option to see what works best for you. Let's say you identified the (A) option mentioned in the above list.

A. When you are alone, maybe straight after meeting a specific person or after specific experiences with a person (e.g., being intimate with your partner, going for lunch with a friend) or when you are in a specific place, e.g. only at or after work, only at home, only when with someone, or straight after being with one specific person.

In this case, it's probably a matter of lack of affection and/or stress from not being able to deal with specific feelings. It's like when you hug someone and you don't receive a hug back - there's a gap that feels like something's missing, there's a pleasure that needs to be fulfilled and that's when we turn to food as a comforter. Food gives you instant gratification. It literally fills up a space in your body and compensates for the emptiness you've experienced.

If you have cravings when you're alone or after meeting specific people or participating in specific events, food serves you as compensation for a lack of pleasure/love/affection that you've experienced. It's as though everyone needs to fill up a *bottle of pleasure* every day. If it isn't filled up by good feelings, pleasurable experiences, or lovely people, it needs to be filled somehow, and the quick fix is food.

A1. What to do?

First of all, ask yourself: 'How can I express how I feel and fill the gap?'

I will give you some examples but I really want you to ask yourself: 'What makes me feel full of pleasure and satisfaction?'

You know within yourself what are those things that make you feel satisfied, and they'll come to you if you ask yourself with an open mind. They can be as little and easy as a manicure, a text, a song, a hug, a kiss, a phone call, or a hot shower.

Here are some examples that can help you find what works for you:

- If it's about a person in particular, address the issue directly, do not linger in negative feelings. If you have a discussion, make sure you resolve the issue instead of leaving it open for the next day or whenever you feel differently. Eliminate the stress as soon as you can and avoid creating the gap in the first place

- If you can't solve the issue straight away or deal with the person that is causing you to experience cravings or look for comfort food, shift your focus immediately to an activity you are sure makes you feel good so that you can fill your pleasure bottle in a different way. This can be taking a hot shower, reading a page from your favourite book, journaling, repeating your affirmations, dancing to your favourite song, writing a gratitude list, or calling a good friend.

- Drink water and breathe very slowly, close your eyes and inhale, then exhale for double the time you've inhaled (e.g. count 1, 2, 3 when you inhale and then 1, 2, 3, 4, 5, 6 when you exhale) and envision a relaxing scene - for me it's a sandy beach and the shoreline with the water slowly coming and going, on a bright day. Even a few minutes of this are effective to create a state of pleasure and relaxation if you immerse yourself completely. Breathing deeply alone automatically brings more oxygen into your brain, which, as a consequence, functions better straight away and helps you make better decisions. I find this one of my most effective tricks because it's so simple. It can be used anytime and anywhere and gives instant comfort!

- If you really feel like you have to put something in your mouth, don't make it look like a bad thing and look for a good snack to satisfy your craving. Remember, the goal and focus here is on filling the pleasure bottle. Instead of choosing something that makes you even more sad or irritable (e.g., sugary snacks that cause negative feelings like guilt, heaviness, OR salty things that dehydrate your body and take away even more energy and good feelings from you), choose something that takes longer to chew and doesn't add any more negative feelings. This can be raw carrots, an apple (that you have to actually bite into), nuts or dried fruit. Eat slowly and chew methodically, so that your brain is well aware that you're eating. At the same time, pick a snack that will make you feel good mentally because you didn't deprive yourself of the pleasure of eating. You are doing the right thing physically because you are ingesting something that's good for your body and doesn't make you gain weight!

B. During specific times of the day, e.g. during the morning or late at night, or in the middle of the night.

If you're experiencing cravings at specific times of the day, this may be due to the fact that you're not eating as frequently as you should or in the right amount. Maybe you skip breakfast and you constantly feel like you want to eat during the late morning. Perhaps you skip dinner or have too light meals during the afternoon and then you wake up in the middle of the night wanting food.

The next sections of this book will be incredibly helpful for this situation, as you'll find the exact tricks and tips to get you to embrace and master the right habits. However, for now, make sure you have small portions often during the day so there are no huge gaps between one meal and the next. Make sure you drink a lot of water to keep yourself hydrated, and also so you don't confuse being hungry with being thirsty.

Also, when you're experiencing those sort of cravings, check how long it's been since your last meal! If it's been more than five hours, you can easily guess why your body wants food. You entered in a sort of starvation mode where your body feels deprived and really hungry and in need of energy!

B1. What to do?

It can be helpful to put an alarm on your phone every four hours, starting from your breakfast, so that you don't go without eating for more than four hours at a time. By eating, I mean even a small snack like a fruit or some nuts, a piece of toast with olive oil, or a few slices of avocado.

The important thing is that you don't let your body enter starvation mode. Aim to have three main meals a day (breakfast, lunch, and dinner) and two or three snacks during the day, and increase your water intake. If you keep your body nourished but light at the same time, this will have a great effect on your metabolism and your energy levels.

C. **When you feel intense emotions, like you are extremely happy, sad, or stressed out, when some particular event happens and you feel overwhelmed or experience strong feelings and emotions**

In this case, food is a quick and easy way to unconsciously process your feelings. You need a physical way to help you process the events and emotions you're experiencing. This is completely normal and quite common. It is referred to as "emotional eating."

Think about going through a break-up. Most people either gain or lose a lot of weight. Sometimes we feel like things are bigger than us and we're overwhelmed. Our mind can't cope with all that's going on, so our body takes over and experiences changes for us.

C1. What to do?

The best thing is to find another way out for you to process whatever is going on. Ask yourself: "What would make me release the excess of happiness/ sadness/ stress/ emotions/ anger?"

Here are some examples:

- Speaking with a special person who can hold space for you and listen, someone you can talk with freely and openly knowing you won't be judged (your parent/ sibling/ best friend/ coach). Describing what's happened will make you express and let out some of the weight of these positive or negative feelings. Have you ever experienced the feeling of being lighter after speaking with someone or revealing a secret? It's the same process! Ever heard the expression: "a weight off my shoulders"? That's the feeling you will achieve.

- Doing something that involves your body. It might be anything from doing some deep cleaning of part of your house, to jumping up and down to your favourite song, to going for a fast walk. Anything that involves your body moving and gets you to do some intense physical activity, even for a few minutes, is a good choice.

- Again, if you feel like you have to put something in your mouth, don't make it feel like a bad thing. Look for healthy food to satisfy your hankering and do you good. You can choose something that makes you "busy." Find a recipe online and start cooking it, or, if you can't wait to eat, choose something that takes a while to chew. Look in the previous section for some ideas of snacks you can have.

D. None of the above, *and* it's always a specific type of food.

In that case, don't despair! If you found yourself not falling into any of the above categories and always craving specific foods, like a particular chocolate bar or a fast-food burger, the next section 2.3.3 is focused precisely on this case.

Chapter Summary

- We examined the reasons why emotional eating is so prevalent.

- Several scenarios were examined where this occurs. We've alked about how best to process these situations in constructive ways.

2.3.3: Food Addictions and How to Heal Them

Chapter Summary

In this chapter, you will learn:

- How easily we can become hooked on the wrong foods.

- Several ways to take your mind and body out of that dependence.

In the next chapter, you will learn:

- The importance of high-fibre foods.

It's been scientifically proven that some foods, usually those with a high content of sugar and salt, can cause real addictions. In the same way some people are addicted to smoking cigarettes, you can be addicted to chocolate cake or fries. In other words, you crave a certain type of food because you've consumed too much of it and your body and brain have become dependent on it. Obviously, it wasn't your intention to get addicted, but it happened. I remember I started eating a specific fast-food very often because we had a problem with our fridge at home and I felt I didn't have much choice. The fast-food place was cheap and close to my house, so it was extremely convenient. And then I found myself addicted to that food.

Your addiction may be even more ingrained due to habits you've grown up with. For example, if babies or toddlers are given two desserts a day, they will be at risk of forming an addiction to sugar later in life. They are the victims in this situation; they have no say in their diet or eating habits.

D1. What to do?

If you think you need to eliminate this food from your life, but the thought of trying causes feelings of discouragement or failure, it's probably because you believe you can't do it or you've tried to before and you couldn't. You'll be happy to know that going cold-turkey is not the only solution, nor, indeed, the best one.

Why? Because as good as it can be to get rid of that food, stopping it from one day to the next can be very unpleasant and have repercussions on your mood and your body. For example, people who consume a lot of sugar, and then quit abruptly, are highly likely to experience migraines, irritability, and even flickering vision, and inability to sleep properly. This means that extremes are not recommended even if you ultimately want to—and will—get rid of your addiction/cravings. Instead of making drastic changes, here's what you can do—decrease your consumption of that specific food by the following methods.

- Trying new things. Switch your mindset to one of an adventurous explorer—there are millions of amazing foods that are delicious and simple to prepare. I bet some of them are easy to find in the shop next door, but you've never tried them. So, look for them, look for new recipes, and search online for healthy recipes. I'm not going to give you examples because the ones I follow may be using ingredients that are not available to you. However, I'm 100% sure you can find plenty of them that use produce available in your country.

- Drink water and breathe deeply, as we've discussed earlier in this book. As simple as it sounds, water hydrates your body and breathing takes more oxygen to your brain. You function better overall, and as a consequence you make better decisions for yourself. It's a positive spiral!

- Put yourself in a position where that specific food is not available to you but make sure you have something else available as a replacement so you don't feel deprived. For instance, don't have biscuits available in your kitchen, in your office, or in your car. Have nuts or fruit or dried fruit at hand, instead.

- When or if you end up having the food that caused your addiction again, don't beat yourself up. Instead, make the decision to forgive yourself. This is both cleansing and empowering. Repeat to yourself: "I forgive you, I love you, and I decide to love you more." Decide to become a better version of you, write down exactly how you feel about it, so you bring awareness to that moment. Also write down how you're determined to feel instead, and how much better your life is when you're finally over this addiction. Write it as though it's already happening and repeat as many affirmations as you can about you being in control, taking the best actions for yourself, and being free, light, and full of energy. Writing things down will inevitably make you much less inclined to eat the food again because your brain is naturally and automatically drawn to what's most pleasurable for you so it will clearly remember the experience.

- Remind yourself that it's absolutely 100% possible to quit addiction, much like smoking and alcohol, so you can beat any kind of food addictions too! It's only a matter of deciding in the first place!

In time, doing something else instead of emotional eating will become your new habit, and you will automatically take a break to relieve your stress in many other ways, instead of eating something that might not be good for you.

Now that we've discussed **Eating**, let's move on to the second **E** in the **S.W.E.E.T. M.A.P.**

Chapter Summary

- We've looked at how we can get accustomed to the wrong foods.

- Cold turkey solutions may work - but they're terribly drastic and often debilitating in the short term.

- Wean yourself off such foods by having alternative recipes, drinking water, journaling and having healthy snacks to hand.

- Don't beat yourself up if you occasionally fall off the wagon! Keep in mind the 80/20 rule.

2.4 E—Exit: How To Make It Easy For Your Body To Get Rid Of What You Don't Need

Chapter Summary

In this chapter, you will learn:

- The value of high-fibre foods.
- Simple foods that help keep you 'regular.'

In the next chapter, you will learn:

- If calorie-counting is *really* a useful exercise?
- About some highly effective tables and trackers I'd love to share with you!

Well, we're going to talk about something we all do and which is a super-simple sign of what's going on in your body. You know, one of the first questions a paediatrician will ask when a new-born comes in for a health check-up in the very first days of his or her life (and even long after) is:

"How are her bowel movements?"

Do you know what this means? You've probably figured it out by now, but to make sure we're clear, I want you to think about how often you go to the toilet to do your serious business. That's because the frequency and quality of your bowel movements are a strong indicator of your health and wellbeing. Let's explore this a little more in depth.

Okay, it's not the most glamorous topic in the world. But, while it may be a bit uncomfortable to talk about, your bowel movements are a great indicator of your overall health. If you struggle to characterise the quality of your bowel movements, there is even a Bristol Stool Chart to help you with that.[30] This way, you can describe your bowel movements using Types 1 to 7.

Also, the next section in this book will help you determine that because it will make it clear to you if things are going okay or if there's work to do. For example, if you find yourself using the bathroom easily every day, that's fine. However, if you notice that you only go once per week, and your weight only increases, you can easily figure out why, and you can give more focus to this aspect of your health. If this is the case for you, no, I don't want you to run to the pharmacy straight away because I've got a story for you about this before you go!

A client of mine was really struggling with bowel movements. He had been struggling for so long that his doctor gave him medication, but even that didn't work. So, I shared my secret with him, which he was very sceptical about, that he nearly laughed in my face when I explained it to him! Nonetheless, he trusted me enough to try. Here it is: as soon as you wake up, relax and sip a glass or a mug of hot water before doing anything or drinking anything else. I know, you don't blame him for laughing! But that is all there is to it! He did it and it worked from day one. Every time he did it, it worked. Months later, he told me that whenever he used this method, it was effective.

Again, food is another excellent helper with bowel frequency, and you can do some simple research about foods that are remarkably beneficial and can be found easily in your area. You'll want to consume high fibre, plant-based foods on a regular basis to regulate the health of your bowel movements— and the best part is, these healthy foods have no negative side effects, and there are so many of them that I'm sure there are many that you'll find delicious!

Just to mention some of my favourites, and the ones that I find really helpful the very few times I find myself constipated (it can always happen—maybe when travelling, or when eating out or at a friend's house), here are some excellent options:

- Plums
- Figs
- Lentils (you can make a delicious lentil soup!)
- Pears
- Strawberries

- Avocados
- Raspberries
- Carrots
- Beets
- Broccoli
- Artichokes
- Brussel sprouts
- Kidney beans
- Split peas
- Quinoa
- Oats
- Popcorn
- Chia seeds
- Coconut
- Pistachios
- Walnuts
- Sweet potatoes
- Yogurt

From this list, select what you like, what you don't like, and what you've never tried. Explore and experiment with your food, make it fun, and reap the benefits. If you want to increase your fibre intake, do it slowly over a period of several days to avoid bloating and gas, and—of course—always drink plenty of water.

The great thing about increasing your fibre intake is that it doesn't just fight constipation. Fibre also benefits other aspects of your health. It feeds friendly bacteria in your gut. It's very good for promoting weight loss and lowering your blood sugar levels. It reduces cholesterol, and helps in reducing the risk of cancer.

Let's move on to the **T** in our **S.W.E.E.T. M.A.P.**

Chapter Summary

- We've looked at our bowels (!) and gained an understanding of how important it is they function efficiently.

- A simple treatment - a mug of hot water, first thing - can be extremely helpful.

- There are a range of easily obtainable high-fibre foods you can utilise and are super beneficial for your health and wellness.

2.5 T- Tracking: The Smartest Way To Lose Weight Without Obsessing Over Numbers (With My Unique Daily Trackers Included!)

Chapter Summary

In this chapter, you will learn about:

- The pitfalls of calorie-counting.

- A super-efficient table to assist you with food intake.

In the next chapter, you will learn:

- The importance of mindfulness to eating and .

I've never been a big fan of numbers. That might be because my parents are both maths teachers, and numbers were our daily bread. Or maybe it's because I've always been fascinated more by feelings and emotions than numbers and science.

Anyway, when it was my time to lose weight, and all I was hearing was, "You need to count your calories!" I would back off before even starting. I knew it wasn't my thing; I also instinctively realised I would have hated it, and it wasn't a practical or realistic approach in my life. Constantly being anxious about my calorie count? And all of those charts and graphs and *numbers*! No, thank you.

Back then, I didn't know much about changing my mindset around my own beliefs. However, I was so determined to keep track of and be able to lose weight *without* using numbers that I found an incredibly simple and effective way that got me, and later on my clients, excellent results without obsessing and stressing over numbers at all.

Sure, there are plenty of apps available now that automatically count your calories, add them up, and tell you how many more or less you need to eat. However, I don't particularly recommend them because of the following reasons:

- The number of calories you are supposed to consume daily is quite variable and depends on many factors that are not *only* your current weight and height. So, as discussed previously, the number provided on the BMI chart is just a rough estimation. It might be completely wrong or pretty far from what your body really needs.

- Forcing yourself to eat more if you haven't met the calorie requirement for a day according to an app or forcing yourself to starve if you've reached your calorie count for the day is both counterproductive and stressful.

It's been proven that the numbers of calories on labels often differ from reality, so the information used would be inaccurate anyway.[33] The U.S. Food and Drug Administration allows a wide latitude—a whopping 20 percent in each direction—to food companies when it comes to calorie counts. What this translates into is that if a label says the food has 200 calories, it could actually have up to 240 or as little as 160, or anything in between. So, based on a 2,000/day calorie diet, or even 1500 calories per day, counting calories doesn't work. Furthermore, there isn't any systematic checking of labels by any oversight organization or committee to see if even that standard is met. The food label accuracy actually lies with the food companies themselves, and is based on the honour system, which anybody could corrupt if they wanted to.

I'm not suggesting that all food companies are liars or anything like that. I'm sure many of them are well-intentioned. But even with a 20 per cent swing in each direction, you won't get an accurate calorie count for the foods you eat in one day, even if you *are* a math wiz!

For another example, there is a short YouTube video about a fantastic guy named Casey Neistat, who added up the calories on the labels of some foods served in common chain restaurants, and then the *actual* calories of the foods.[44] He bought some food items, and then got them analysed in a food lab and here's what he found. After hanging out with some food scientists who used specific tools (like a machine called a

Calorimeter), and did a lot of math, they found out that one banana nut yoghurt muffin has a whopping 740 calories! In fact, all of the foods analysed had *more* calories than were reported by the food manufacturer. It does all tend to strongly indicate that calorie counting is not a great way to go.

Last but not least, numbers can become an obsession. If you think about a lot of eating disorders, numbers are a big part of them: numbers of steps, numbers of reps when exercising, numbers on the scale, numbers of calories, and so on. This is a big reason why I don't recommend calorie counting—because there's the potential there for number counting to become a compulsive obsession that can dominate your life. Even if it's done for the best of reasons, it can still turn into a borderline neurosis that is ultimately self-defeating.

However, in case you actually love numbers, are very numbers-oriented, and are using an app to count calories—or you would like to start using one—don't panic. I'm not going to tell you that you need to stop. I just want you to be aware of and not rely on those numbers as though they're always correct and completely factual. Instead, use them as an *estimation* without getting overly preoccupied with them.

That said, keeping track of *what* you eat is essential, and it is one of the most effective things you can do to actually lose weight fast and naturally!

So how do you do it without counting calories?

Can you write? Can you type? If the answer is yes, you just need to use the table below every single day and you're done. Yes, it's as simple as writing or typing some notes every day, but there's more behind it than that, and it is a truly valuable tool. Here's how it works and what you can expect from using my daily trackers designed specifically for this purpose.

You will be:

- Eating less

- Enjoying your food more

- Feeling better

- Appreciating yourself more

- More connected with your body

- Losing weight

- Improving the quality of your life

You'll be doing all this nearly effortlessly!

You will become aware of what's going on with your eating habits because your brain will need to give your diet more attention in terms of time and intensity.

It will be easier to switch gears and implement the right habits when you track them on paper (or on your phone or laptop—

connect with me on social for the editable pdf. version) because you'll easily visualise what's going wrong—and how to fix it.

- For example, you'll know immediately if you're not eating enough, or if you're eating at the wrong times, or if you're eating the wrong portions. All of these are potential blocks to your weight loss and your wellbeing and you'll quickly be able to identify them because the visual aspect of the tracker will make it very clear to you.

- You'll be naturally inclined to eat less and be more mindful about what you eat because you know you have to write it down and notice both what you eat and how you feel, which means facing it on all levels. You'll experience genuine and effortless weight loss.

- You'll experience a general increase in the quality of your mindset, your mood, your energy levels, and your feelings. Your weight will start decreasing in no time.

Find the link below to access the table, and make sure you read this section to find out how to get the most out of it.

Here's the printable version I share with my clients. You're welcome! If you want to find out more about trackers—I have a wide variety of trackers, including daily wellness and shopping lists and meal plans that are in printable versions or editable

pdf. files—feel free to reach out on social media, I'd be very happy to share them with you!
http://bit.ly/juliastrackers

Using this tracker, and visualising the different boxes, will make you aware of your habits and how to adjust them.

- For example, regarding eating, if you find the "extra" box full and larger than you're comfortable with, increase the quantities of your main meals, and see if you can get rid of some extras.

- If you find that three out of the six boxes are empty, you can go and regulate your times and portions so you can increase the number of your meals while decreasing the quantities.

- You'll soon realise how much easier it is to change your habits when you have clarity, you have everything written down in front of you, and you are actively involved.

Chapter Summary

- Calorie counting sounds terribly scientific, but it doesn't take into account all sorts of variables, and it's often based on unreliable information supplied by the food manufacturers.

- Tracking (without numbers) is extremely important to become more aware of what's going on with our food and eating patterns, and optimise them.

- Feel free to access and use my daily trackers - they're proven and they work!

M.A.P.

2.6 M—Mindfulness: How To Lose Weight And Live The Happy Way!

Chapter Summary

In this chapter, you will learn:

- Just how vital mindful eating is for many reasons.
- How to put this theory into practice.

In the next chapter, you will learn:

- The tremendous benefits of physical activity for, not only weight loss, but your general mental and physical health and simple ways to stay active if you're not a fan of the gym.

Most of us have heard the word "mindfulness," but what does it mean?

Mindfulness is defined by Oxford Languages as:

"A mental state achieved by focusing one's awareness on the present moment, while calmly acknowledging and accepting one's feelings, thoughts, and bodily sensations, used as a therapeutic technique."[45]

Sounds interesting, but how does that translate into the way we behave around food?

Well, think about how many times it has happened to you that you had your meal or snack while watching a movie, or in front of your laptop or TV (or another screen), or talking with someone on the phone, or while working, and doing another million things at the same time?

And then, when you were left with an empty plate or an empty food wrapping paper, you felt like you didn't even eat, and you'd like to start over with your meal?

Most likely, that happened *not* because your stomach wasn't full at the end, but instead because *your mind was too busy elsewhere to register the process of you eating,* and therefore, missed out on the natural pleasure of eating.

You see, eating is meant to be a pleasure; when you eat, both your mind and your body expect to experience pleasure. This is why eating activates the pleasure centres in the brain. If one of them is missing out on its part, there's a void that needs to be filled.

If I asked you, "What did you eat for lunch yesterday?" would you even remember?

Of course, life is so fast and so crazy busy that often we forget to eat, don't eat well, or don't care what we consume. However, if you think about it, eating should really be one of the top priorities in life, because hey, you know—we can't last long without nourishing ourselves!

I'd like to bring up new-borns again, maybe because my two little boys have taught me so much about life in such a short time. Nonetheless, this is a simple core fact. As soon as a new-born is out in the world and is placed on their mother's chest, they open their mouth and move their head towards the breast and look to feed themselves.

After *breathing*, the second most important thing is *eating*; a new-born baby, who's helpless, can't talk, can't move much, and can't do anything really, is born with the instinct to eat and the necessary skills to make it happen—right after birth! If you don't have experience with a new-born, trust me, it's amazing to see how tiny and helpless humans can be, yet they are so determined and persistent in looking for food.

Don't forget about the phase where all babies do is put everything into their mouths just for the pleasure of tasting, and trying, and discovering new things. Or, when they start eating solid foods, and they have a fantastic time experiencing new tastes—by grabbing food and putting it all over their hands and faces (if their parents are like me and let them enjoy the experience!)

So, this whole story points out and underlines the fact that eating is not only a duty, a right, a natural instinct, and an absolute priority, but it's also a *pleasure* by definition.

Food is your friend, it wants the best for you. It's there to make your life better, to make you stronger, to make you more beautiful, and to help you be happier. Having a beautiful, peaceful, healthy, pleasurable relationship with food is an asset that can improve your life by a lot.

What is mindful eating?

Here's a list of the essential things to know about mindful eating, with a particular weight loss perspective:

- Appreciate the food that you eat and the fact that you are eating. It doesn't take long to say thank you and feel grateful, but it does make a huge difference in how you approach food, which helps greatly with losing weight and being at peace with your body.

- Eat slowly because it will not only make you full faster, but it will also satisfy the *mental* part of eating, as well as assisting with digestion.

- Think about eating as a massage: you wouldn't rush it, you would take your time, and you would truly and thoroughly enjoy it. You are worthy of this.

- Don't multitask while you eat. Try to focus on what you're eating and enjoy it as much as possible. If you always complain about not having time to stop for a second and relax, eating is the perfect excuse to do just that. *And* you can have that opportunity multiple times per day, every single day.

- Set boundaries *for* yourself and make them non-negotiable.

- Really slow down and listen to your body.

- Be grateful and embrace the amazing journey you're on.

- Celebrate every meal, and every good feeling you get from eating, every step of the way!

- Always keep in mind that everything you do or you want to do comes from a place of *love*—*love* for yourself, *love* for your life, *love* for the people who care about you, *love* for your future, and *love* for *love*!

Onward, to the **A** of our **S.W.E.E.T. M.A.P.**

Chapter Summary

- We've looked at mindfulness and eating.

- Take time to appreciate your food - don't multitask when you're having a meal. Enjoy the experience and it will produce much more healthy results.

2.7 A - Activity: How To Stay Active If You're A Sofa Lover (Like Me)

Chapter Summary

In this chapter, you will learn:

- How to examine and offset excuses about avoiding exercise.

- That short bursts of exercise are just as good as prolonged sessions.

- How to make it fun!

In the next chapter, you will learn:

- Self care - for you and those around you.

Having a great balance in how and what you eat is already an incredible help, not only for an easy, sustainable, significant weight loss, but also for your general wellbeing, your positive mood, your energy levels, your performance, and your relationships. However, if you want to get things moving quickly, and uplevel even more with your weight loss and your general wellness, **being physically active** will certainly accomplish that. In this section, you'll find ways to burn extra calories and be fit and healthy with all the benefits this brings, without spending a ton of money or time on gym memberships or exercising all day long.

The Basics:

I was never a sporty girl, and the hours of P.E. at school were my least favourite. I would find any excuse to avoid them! So, when I put on extra weight, the idea of going to a gym—or doing any sort of exercise—scared me a lot. To be honest, I didn't even try.

Nonetheless, I was determined to lose weight, so I researched and experimented as much as I could, and not only was I able to lose weight, but somehow I started to enjoy the benefits of being active. This got me into running and swimming—both of which I now enjoy!

I find both swimming and running to be an amazing way to completely release any negative energy. Moreover, they're relaxing, and they make me feel energetic and positive.

Now, I don't want you to think that I became a marathon runner or an Olympian swimmer, nor that I train every day— or even every week.

When I run, I don't run for more than an hour. When I swim, I swim for about 40 minutes, and trust me, I don't swim fast! I don't go running more than once a week and I do skip some weeks. I haven't been swimming since early 2020 because of Covid, so it's definitely been a while.

However, it's *how* I do those things that counts. I am happy, I am excited, I am looking forward to them, which—as you can imagine—*is a complete game changer!* Again, it was all about my mindset, my self-limiting beliefs, and my lack of confidence.

I had thoughts running around in my head that went something like this:

- "I'm not good at sports."

- "I'm too skinny to do that."

- "I'm too fat to do that."

- "I'm too short to do that."

- "I'm not strong enough for that."

- "What will my friends think about me if I do that?"

- "It's too hard."

- "It's too expensive."

- "It's too far."

- "I don't feel good."

- "As soon as this happens I'll start."

- "I'll start tomorrow or, better still, next week…"

Sound familiar?

These were excuses that I would come up with to avoid even starting *anything* that included exercise. If you find yourself thinking those things, I want you to recognise that they are excuses, and a form of self-sabotage. The latter mainly comes from **fear**: You might be scared of your own reactions or what people will think about you. You might feel very self-conscious and apprehensive about the whole thing because you're going to have to start at the beginning.

Instead, think about it this way. What are your excuses and fears? What, precisely, are your limiting beliefs? Acknowledge them and make some new decisions.

DECIDE that you are stronger, the new you is better, you love the new you, and that nothing, and, I repeat, *nothing* can stop you from becoming the most stunning, confident, and beautiful woman or man that you are meant to be!

That said, I don't want you to change everything drastically today because that doesn't work long term. You're not here for a quick fix, but for a _real long-lasting solution_. So, what you need to focus on is a few simple steps every single day!

In this next section, you'll find extremely simple, free, and enjoyable ways that you can effortlessly incorporate into your daily life to be more active. You will also be getting your body to move more every day, so that you'll lose weight and feel far better—_without_ stressing out or being in pain. Then, if you're ready to take it to the next step—being active and its benefits are addictive, in a good way—chances are, you will want to uplevel in that area too! However, that's up to you. You'll have the basics in place that will get you results _without_ needing to go to extremes.

So, to sum up the basics before action time:

- Recognise your excuses and stop making them. You're stronger than them.

- Work on your mindset to rewrite your story; go from "I am lazy" to "I want to be fit and can do this."

- Remember that the past only has the power you _let_ it have on you.

- Decide that the present and the future are yours to shape.

- Affirm that you're an amazing, incredible, courageous, and powerful person and you're worthy simply because you are a human being on this earth.

- Embrace the best lifestyle for you and be kind to yourself.

Don't forget that I believe in you. You've got this!

Action time

- Make a list of your favourite excuses; writing them down will help you debunk them and approach them from a different angle next time you come across them.

- Make sure your new beliefs are in place, and you remind yourself of them daily.

For example:

- "It's becoming very easy for me to stay active every day."

- "I love staying active, and I feel better and better every day."

- "My new lifestyle is amazing, and makes me feel more at peace and beautiful every day."

- "I love improving my mindset and my body every day!"

Make sure that your new beliefs are something along those lines that ensure that you feel amazing on a daily basis. Make a list of new decisions, intentions, and commitments. Experiment with all the ways to stay active daily. You can write down your personal list and pick and choose from that on a daily basis. A good idea is to give each new activity one or more stars according to how much you enjoyed it. The reason for that is so your mind acknowledges and is aware of how great you feel—and automatically moves you towards experiencing more of that feeling.

You don't necessarily have to work out for 30 minutes in one shot to reap the benefits of exercise. Studies have shown that short bursts of activity throughout the day can be just as effective as long periods of exercise. If you're looking for evidence, there's a 2018 health news article called, "*Short bursts of Exercise as Beneficial for Health as Longer Workouts, Study Finds,*" published by the Independent newspaper.[46] This study proved once and for all that however you get your NHS-recommended 150 minutes of exercise per week, it always has a positive impact on your health. Short, 30-minute bursts of activity several times per week even reduces mortality rates from all causes.

So, there you go: The "I don't have time!" excuse is now void!

Some of my favourite, most effective ways to stay active are done while I'm having fun. They are 100% free and take literally no more than 10 minutes. I don't need special clothes, equipment, money, or even to go out of my house.

If you've got kids or a partner, or one of your friends that are on the same kind of weight loss journey, you can have them join in the fun with you, and trust me—you'll have a great time together. And remember: having fun sends signals to your brain that you're feeling really *GOOD!* Your brain will look for that reward again and again, and will make you want to experience it more often.

Let's talk a bit about dancing. YouTube has a whole bunch of salsa and Zumba dance videos that are terrific to dance along to, allowing you to get your exercise every day in a fun way. Dancing is good for you, and there are tons of different types— there's also hip hop, ballroom, club dancing, and ballet. The possibilities are endless.

According to WebMD, a 30 minute dance class can burn between 130 and 250 calories, and that's approximately the same amount as jogging.[47] Now, I don't know about you, but I prefer dancing to jogging.

There are other benefits to dancing, like the fact that it can make you stronger and better coordinated and it's good for your heart. Dancing to choreographed work is also good for your brain since it requires you to memorise several different moves in a sequence. Dancing is aerobic exercise and increases your flexibility as well. It targets your core, your glutes, your arms and legs, and strengthens your back. It's also generally low-impact. If you're following along with a YouTube video, dancing is free and you can do it in your home. It's also beneficial for your mental health.

The music alone makes you want to move. There are classes that are just three minutes long. Initially, it will probably take you twice the time to have fun figuring out how to repeat the movements. Simply by doing a dance sequence twice, you'll burn many calories and activate many muscles. Imagine how good and satisfied you'll feel afterwards!!

There are endless playlists for you to have fun with, especially if you love Latin American music like I do! If you prefer another kind of music, simply type into YouTube your favourite style of music and keywords like: workout, training, Zumba, and so on.

You can dance when you get back from work to release stress, and it works like magic. You can also break into a little dance in other circumstances, too.

- While you wait for your meal to be ready for dinner, so that you avoid snacking and spoiling your meal.

- You can dance as soon as you wake up in the morning in order to wake up in a great mood.

- Dance when you're bored instead of going to your fridge!

- You can use dancing as a challenging game with whoever you want to have a fun time with—your partner, your kids, and your friend or neighbour. For instance, see who can dance a choreographed dance without a mistake, and then the one who loses has to run around the house or jump up and down 10 times.

Alternatively, there are also plain workouts on YouTube that don't involve dancing, but are very diverse and come in all types. You can find several that you like the most and bookmark the web pages that they're on, so that you can return to them easily whenever you want. Some workouts are perfect to be active and work your entire body in less than 10 minutes.

There's every kind of workout—short, long, for the upper body, for the lower body, with explanations, without explanations, with or without music, focused on specific parts of your body, and so on. All you need to do is look for them on YouTube. Make sure the trainer in the video is authentic and the training serves your purpose, and you're all set for a fun workout.

When you look at the amazing bodies of the dancers and aerobics instructors, I want you to think that's you. I want you to feel fantastic and to believe you have all you need to look like them. This doesn't mean that you have to get to that level of fitness or that exact body shape. I'm nowhere near that myself because that's not what I even want. I just want to have energy, feel great, and have a healthy body. But knowing that everything is possible for you will help you get rid of any possible jealousy, envy, and other negative feelings you may feel.

Remember to never compare yourself with others because there's no sense in comparing someone's starting point to someone's else's middle or end point. Aim to have fun experimenting with some short training, find out what you like, including music, and include your workout in your daily or weekly routine. Never forget the power of one song! Put your headphones on—I have bluetooth headphones with noise cancellation, and they're great! Put them on and put your favourite song on. Dance, jump, and kick back and forth. Yes, even right now!

Dance like one person is watching—the person who loves you exactly the way you are, the person who knows everything about you, and *loves you anyway.* Perhaps you think that person doesn't exist, and that's okay—it's not your parents, it's not your best friend, it's not even your partner. ***Because that person can be you.*** Only *you* know everything about yourself, only *you* know what you've been through, only *you* know what you've experienced, and only *you* know your deepest desires. Love yourself for *who you are.*

At the end of the day, what is love? Feeling deep affection for something or someone no matter their imperfections. You don't need to be perfect to be loved, you need to accept yourself. That's the starting point for whatever change you want to make. There's absolutely no better gift that you can give yourself than that.

And this might be the single most powerful thing you'll ever do for yourself.

Don't forget to add your music and dance routine to your "Daily Magic Track Table!"

On top of all of this, make sure you value, celebrate, and keep track of *everything* that keeps your body active on a daily basis, including things like:

- Cleaning the house.

- Cooking your own food.

- Walking your dog.

- Parking farther away than you normally do when you go shopping instead of looking for the closest car park.

- Taking the stairs instead of the lift every single time.

- Tracking your steps with an app on your phone, a pedometer, or a smartwatch.

Again, write it all down, and you'll see how easy it is to fill up the **ACTIVITY** column in your table. You'll feel much better about yourself for doing something good for you every day.

Also, explore ways to be active when you would normally be sitting down. For example, instead of seeing a friend at a coffee place for a chat, grab your drink and invite them for a walk instead. Do something that involves moving your body while watching TV. For example, choose some light arm or leg exercises, and do them alternately while watching your favourite show. While you're on the phone, simply walk around your home, get up from your desk and walk while talking. It's crazy how super-simple, easy switches in your daily life can make a difference in your weight loss and wellbeing.

Every time you're uncertain, tired, stressed or unmotivated, think about this: simply by moving your body *A LITTLE BIT,* you'll gain energy, be able to refocus, and reduce your stress levels. You really don't need crazy exercising or long hours. It's seriously not hard and it's totally worth it, trust me that I am not sporty at all and still have easily kept my weight off for more than ten years now, while eating food I love and staying active using the exact methods I shared with you in this chapter.

Fully celebrate and acknowledge the benefits you're experiencing, and celebrate how amazing you are being to yourself—trust me—you won't be able to stop, *and* you'll get a body you love in no time. It'll be beyond your wildest dreams!

Let's move on to the **P** in our **S.W.E.E.T. M.A.P.**

Chapter Summary

- Physical activity can come in all varieties and has been medically and scientifically proven to be enormously beneficial.

- Check out YouTube as a great source of exercise and dance videos.

- Work with a friend or just let yourself go on your own!

2.8 P - Priority:
You Matter—All the Time

Chapter Summary

In this chapter, you will learn:

- There's little to be gained by ignoring your own health, either mentally or physically.

- Ensure you make time for yourself to relax and gather strength.

- Organise your days in advance.

In the next chapter, you will learn:

- The damage caused by negative spirals - and how to conquer them.

Remember, you want to lose weight without pain, without it being so hard, and, especially, without getting all the weight back and seeing all your productive work vanish. To do this, you need to make yourself, your health, and your overall wellbeing a priority. You also need to make the decision to feel good about this a priority because this will help you as a person and have a positive impact in all areas of your life.

Prioritising yourself, your health, and your wellbeing will also have a good effect on your loved ones, so this is a valuable way to make it happen! Once you've embraced a lifestyle that you simply *LOVE* and it does you good in all aspects—for both your mindset and your body—it will be beneficial not only for you but for those around you.

Your health and wellbeing are probably the most valuable assets in your life. You cannot pour from an empty cup. You have to be whole, full, at peace with yourself to be a positive force in other people's lives.

This is not selfish, this is self-care, which is not synonymous with self-indulgence or being self-centred. Self-care is taking care of yourself so that you can be healthy and whole, you can do your job and be an active and positive part of your family. By doing this, you will set a good example for your children and peers.

Anxiety and depression are real things that may affect us all at some point in our lives, but when you practice self-care and do it on a daily basis, you can conquer these states of being. We cope better with stress when we look after ourselves.

Think about this. Kelsey Patel, author and wellness expert, says, *"People are feeling lonelier and less able to unwind and slow down, which makes them feel more anxious and overwhelmed by even the simplest tasks.*"[48] Some experts believe that in this era, we have entered an epidemic of anxiety and depression. And it's not accidental that the coaching industry is growing at light speed, everyone of us needs a safe space to be and grow, and the right coach for you, the one that's aligned with your values and desires, can give you exactly that: a safe space where you are seen, listened to without being judged, can be yourself, can heal, can grow. All my clients, and also myself with my own coaches, have accelerated our growth and elevated our quality of life literally in weeks and while feeling very safe and held and seen. I truly love and value every single one of my clients and their journey, and I feel so blessed to be doing this job that I adore. I could probably write another entire book on that, but for now let's move to some other very useful tools for you.

So, how best to practice self-care, and what does it mean, specifically?

The World Health Organization states that self-care is "*the ability of individuals, families, and communities to promote health, prevent disease, maintain health, and to cope with illness and disability with or without the support of a healthcare provider.*"[49]

Self-care isn't merely about reducing your stress levels. It will improve your immune system and self-esteem too - that's what researchers have found. Self-care will make you more productive at work, as well.

Therefore, if you like yoga, go to town when you practice it! Some people recommend meditation, and there are many ways that you can practice guided meditation available online. With guided meditation, you will listen to soothing, soft music while you relax your body and mind and take deep breaths.

There are endless ways to prepare healthy meals that are delicious. It doesn't have to always be broccoli soup! Actually, my next book is all about meal planning in a fun way and includes tons of super-healthy, easy, and tasty recipes. Keep an eye out for it.

Other forms of self-care can be spending time in nature or setting time to be away from all electronics and screens. This is time to focus on you and the benefits are great. You *do* have time to do this, trust me.

When we are striving to reach a focused place where we are promoting our own health, managing any problems that arise, and preventing illnesses we can, keeps us at a place biologists call "homeostasis," which essentially means that we are balanced.

Practising self-care is as much about coping strategies as it is about being healthy. Sometimes, people who are generally self-sacrificial, women in particular, need to be convinced to practice self-care. If you're one of these people, acknowledge that self-care is extremely important and open up to ways self-care can improve your health and life. For example, it will help you live, work, and function at your absolute best. How you practice self-care is unique to you. It can be something practical, spiritual, physical, intellectual, or something that you need to get done to relieve tension and feel calm. You are worthy because you are. That's all there is to it.

Remember to always be adaptable and flexible. Your self-care activities right now may be very different from your self-care routine three years from now. Adapt, evolve, and continue to grow. There's no limit to self-improvement. There are always higher goals to reach that will better you. We should be always reaching higher and looking for even better ways of being and living but never forget to appreciate the present moment and what's already here. When you accomplish your weight loss goals, you will still be growing into yourself intellectually and maybe even spiritually, becoming more whole and grounded. This will lead to a more settled, less anxious, and more contented and happy you.

Anything that feels nourishing and nurturing to you can be self-care. That might be scheduling a bath with candles and crystals every two or three days. It might be having a dance-off with your children. Reading that book that you've been meaning to read for ages is also self-care, as is video chatting with your best friends, or—even better—having them over for some quality time.

What nourishes your soul?

Think about the good stuff, when you feel the warm fuzzy feelings inside, and you feel happy, content, and cared for. Then do what makes you feel that way on a regular basis, like it's part of your everyday routine.

Pencil yourself in. Show up for yourself in a way that no one else can. Only *you* know what makes you feel the absolute best feelings. Maybe it's going to the park and listening to children laugh. It could be throwing a ball for your dog to race after and return. Maybe it's lying on the floor and blasting Beethoven's *9th Symphony* or "Despacito." Whatever it is—do it, and do it regularly.

Another simple, yet extremely effective, strategy for being more present and intentional with our time so we can get more of what we want out of it, is to plan tomorrow today. Since implementing this easy, no-fuss life hack, my life has completely changed for the better and what my clients tell me when implementing this, is that the hours in their day seem to multiply instead of vanishing like before! You won't believe what a difference it will make in your daily life until you test it yourself. It works like this:

Write down on a notepad or on your google calendar your hourly schedule for the next day, including what you've got planned, and what you want to make sure you get done. Also add a section for notes and write in there anything that motivates you, that you find relevant or useful so your brain will remember it.

It looks something like this—I'll use mine as an example, but you can make your version:

- 7am-8am Wake up, breakfast with the family, get kids ready for school.

- 8am-9am Get ready for the day, tidy up the kitchen and workspace, take kids to school.

- 9am-10am Journal, check email, check messages, tea, and snack.

- 10am-11am 1:1 client call

- 11am-12pm Send client session notes and reply to emails.

- 12pm-13pm Lunch break.

- 13pm-14pm 1:1 client call

- 14pm-15pm Send client session notes and work on project x.

- 15pm-16pm Pick up kids from school.

- 16pm-17pm Play and be present with kids (outdoors whenever possible), snack.

- 17pm-18pm Family time, prepare dinner.

- 18pm-19pm Dinner + family time.

- 19pm-20pm Bedtime routine.

- 20pm-21pm Reading.

- 21pm-22pm Reading and sleep time.

NOTES:

- Focus!

- You don't need a magic pill!

- You *are* the magic pill!

- Keep forward thinking.

That's just an example of one of my days, as some things are recurring every day, like my meals and journaling. Others are weekly occurrences, like my one-on-one coaching for clients. I do this for every working day and it's magic! Plus, I like to write in the notes the things that I found useful, the things that I learned, and quotes I came across that I liked.

You will be surprised at how much time you have, and how easy it is to include important and pleasurable things into your day when you write them all down. On the flip side, you'll also notice how hard it becomes to procrastinate and get off track when you have such a simple, clear, and straightforward plan!

But if you *still* somehow find ways to self-sabotage, do these simple, easy tricks until your planning becomes a habit:

- Put alarms on your phone.

- Share your plan with someone to keep yourself accountable.

- Find a way *IN ADVANCE* to prevent you from getting off track because prevention is always better than trying to find a cure.

For example:

- If you find your mindset to be negative and you self-sabotage and impede your progress, include mindset work and affirmations into tomorrow's plan.

- If you find yourself not knowing what to eat, plan some food shopping and meal ideas—I have a unique plan that works wonders for me and has made me save a lot of money, time, and stress since I started implementing it a couple of years ago. Connect with me on social media or email me to pre-order my new book about my no-stress meal plan method; it also includes 36 easy, healthy, delicious recipes!

- If you find yourself not including ways to be active, and you have a free hour, make sure you include something that makes you active, even if it's just doing some extra cleaning or going to see a friend for a walk.

You get the point! Visualising it, and having to consciously plan your days, will get you into being organised, exploring your options, quitting your excuses, and making sure you take care of your wellbeing in *all* aspects—which will get you into your positive spiral!

Chapter Summary

- Self care isn't selfishness. By looking after yourself, you're happier, more effective, and more able to help others.

- We've studied the importance of planning your days in advance to get the best out of your time

SECTION 3: COMPOUNDING YOUR WINS

Putting it All Together

By now, you have all the most important pieces in place, and if you've been putting them in practice, I'll bet you're already seeing and experiencing some results. However, I want to add a little icing on the cake to make you take action if you haven't already, and help you to keep it up if you're just starting. In this third section, I will share with you how to compound your success, make your improvements consistent, and truly embody the new confident person you're becoming.

3.1 The Positive Spiral And How To Step Into It

Chapter Summary

In this chapter, you will learn:

- What the positive spiral is, and how it will benefit you.

- How to break free from negative spirals and enter positive ones.

- What *Nulla Dies Sine Linea* means, and how to apply it to your life.

In the next chapter, you will learn:

- How tiny changes are often all it takes.

I'm sure you've experienced negative spirals in your life, those patterns of behaviour often called vicious circles where each step drags you down. They can be food addictions, or habits of self-sabotaging, or self-limiting beliefs.

You think you're fat and you can't control yourself around food—you feel bad and you eat junk food—you gain even more weight—you feel like you can't control yourself around food—you buy more junk food—you gain more weight.

You know how hard it is to break these habits, to act differently, and to get out of that spiral. That's the nature of being in a spiral. You're in this circle where you're so used to certain things that it's really hard to go in a different direction, no matter how much you want it.

However, here's the key to your success—if you enter a *positive spiral* instead of a negative one, it will be just as hard to get out of. Moreover, you won't *want* to get out of it, which will make it even harder for you to stop the amazing things you're doing for yourself.

This is why you need to *consciously create* a virtuous circle, or *positive spiral*, that you truly enjoy every single day. This positive spiral is such that you in your entirety—body and mind—will love it and benefit from it. The initial steps can be difficult, but then that's the case with most things - getting started. Don't worry about it at all - I'm going to help you with that.

There are two main tricks to shift from a negative to a positive spiral.

1. Make a list of possible negative spiral breakers. These are things that, as a matter of fact, have an indisputably positive impact on you and can automatically shift your mood. They make you feel good or laugh, even for no reason. As much as I can't say what exactly will make *you* enter *your* positive spiral because I don't know what makes *you* happy, and what makes *you* feel great, I can tell you what works for me. I love things like:

- Reading

- Travelling

- Sandy beaches

- Talking with my sister and my mum

- Journaling a list of things I'm grateful for

- Visualising my goals

- Going for a walk with my husband and kids

- Thinking about when we'll get our first dog

- Planning my next work projects

- Working with my clients

- Watching a clip of *The Ellen Show or The Late Late Show with James Corden*

Any time I am doing one of those things, I know for a fact that my mood improves just because I did them. Make sure you make your own list, maybe you love the mountains and don't even have siblings!

2. Establish new routines. Remember, so much of what we've covered in this book is about habits. It takes approximately 30 days to form a habit. This is why my programmes start from 6 weeks, which is the right time to learn and start implementing routines consistently. To find out more about my programmes and how you can get personalised support to achieve your goals, please connect me directly on social media.

3. What you focus on expands, so always concentrate on progress and accomplishments, celebrating your steps forward even if they're tiny ones. This will move you forward. Always be kind with yourself and observe yourself like you're watching your most precious treasure. For example, you notice you're in a negative spiral and you're sabotaging your progress. Instead of feeling bad or telling yourself you're not good enough and you've fallen off the wagon again, think:

- Would I be telling this to my child? (If you have children, otherwise you can use whoever you love the most, like your friend, a special relative, or your partner.)

- What would I tell them?

- What can I do to shift into a positive spiral? Start with small things like your positive spiral list from above.

Never underestimate the power of one simple action or one simple laugh; they can change your entire world!

Chapter Summary

- Negative spirals make us feel trapped - so you escape from them by replacing them with positive ones.

- List the things that make you happy, establish routines around them and always focus on progress.

3.2: *Nulla Dies Sine Linea* = No Day Without A Line

Chapter Summary

In this chapter, you will learn:

- The value of incremental improvements.

In the next chapter, you will learn:

- Some brilliant and easy ways to boost your self-confidence.

The above is one of my favourite quotes. It is attributed to Apelles, who was a revered painter of the 4th century BC. What this meant was that the painter would never go one day without at least drawing the outline of a picture, no matter how busy he was. What it means for us, on this journey, is that we do not have to change by enormous leaps and bounds. We can change in small, subtle ways that add up to a large overall alteration, but we must practice our small changes every day in order to persevere and keep them fresh in our minds. We must practice diligent perseverance, as Anthony Trollope, the great Nineteenth Century writer, said in his autobiography when referencing this very quote.(49) A diligent perseverance means chipping away and replacing old habits with new ones, and practising them every single day. Trollope added that we do not need to be slaves to our work (or our lifestyle changes), but we do need to keep them at the forefront of our minds, so that they're permanent and lasting changes.

What I love about the Apelles quote is the last word. '*a line*'. He didn't insist that you had to do a full painting every day (he would leave that for Vincent Van Gogh!) What I infer from his advice is that regular, routine practice will have its effect. When you draw that one line every day, then you are making forward progress:

- Maybe it's drinking enough water today.

- It could be going for a walk and actually enjoying it.

- It's appreciating and making peace with a single thing about yourself or about your past today.

- Possibly it's one meal done right that makes you feel light now.

- Maybe it's the one empowering or kind thought that finally pops up into your mind while you are looking in the mirror.

One step at a time, day after day. That's all it takes to see and experience change. That's all it takes to make it happen. No matter how small the changes you are making are, they are still adding up to significant shifts in your overall perspective and lifestyle habits. That's no mean feat and it shouldn't be undervalued.

We also need to acknowledge that celebrating our accomplishments and rewarding ourselves for them are both very important. As human beings, we are always looking for approval, external rewards forge connections in our brains that complete the dopamine-reward circuit. That makes us more and more motivated to keep up with the changes and repeat them over and over again.

Be kind to yourselves, and reward your good behaviour. Positive reinforcement works wonders on adult human beings too, but since we have nobody teaching us what to do, we have to take on the important task of rewarding ourselves. This is so important!

When you set your mind to something, there is literally nothing that you cannot do. So, focus on smaller tweaks to your habits and routines, which will definitely add up to a rewarding change in your outlook, and then in your body. The main focus is always going to be quality not quantity. Quantity will take care of itself if we are practising quality work in our lifestyle changes.

Chapter Summary

- A small amount of constructive work every day is far better than trying to do too much and being overwhelmed.

- Reward yourself for those little steps. Each one will help you travel a long way.

3.3 How to Double Down on Your Self-Confidence

Chapter Summary

In this chapter, you will learn:

- How to be a lion, even if you used to be a dormouse!

There are so many misconceptions about self-confidence. Many people think you're born with it or you're not. Others think you are automatically self-confident when you have certain features, such as a fit body or a high level position in your career.

I think it's a skill. And, like all skills, it can be learnt and developed. Why do I believe this? Because I was the embodiment of the opposite of self-confidence. I was the smallest and shyest girl in the class, I was terribly afraid to speak in front of people, and everybody ignored me because I could not bring myself to talk to them. Fast forward to now, I go live on Facebook and I have conversations with new people nearly every day, I even wrote a book, wow. All I feel is excitement and happiness!

According to dictionaries, self-confidence is a feeling of trust in one's abilities, qualities, and judgement. Working on myself and with my clients, I found the main reason why we don't feel confident and I discovered a practice that can greatly increase self-trust. It's the single most powerful thing that made me evolve from an invisible ghost to a person who has a voice and inspires others. I've tried it on myself and it's worked wonders. My clients have also applied it and it has changed their world, so I'm going to share it with you as well. It's a simple two-step process:

1. **Understand** that the main reason why we don't feel confident is because we focus our attention on what we don't have. We think about what we don't have enough of, what's missing in our lives, what we are not, what we haven't yet accomplished, what we've done wrong, and all the times we believe we made the wrong choice, made the wrong decision, and took the wrong turn. This is what I call a lack mindset and disempowering approach, which is very common.

2. **Consciously shift** the attention to things that improve your confidence. I always ask my clients to make lists because our brain is like a search engine. Your brain will take your input and will respond with an output accordingly. If you type on Google "cute dog", you will get results about cute dogs. If you type "horror story", it will come up with horror stories. So, intentionally prompt your mind to find the good and you'll get the good.

3. To help you here, I'll share one of the exercises that I regularly give to my clients, which is all about getting your brain to come up with the good stuff about you and focus on that to boost confidence. It's simple but super effective.

- All the things you've already accomplished and you're proud of.

- The experiences that got you to become good at something.

- The knowledge you have about certain topics.

- All the obstacles you've overcome.

- The craziness you survived.

- How much good stuff you've already done in this world.

Also, I'll give you some example here of my real life of how this whole process of shifting from disempowering and confidence lowering focus towards an empowering and confidence increasing one here so you can see how powerful this process is:

Considering my body, disempowering thoughts that decrease my confidence are: *My body is not great because of my very visible stretch marks and loose skin. I/my body wasn't able to deliver my kids naturally and without complications (for reference, I dreamed about a natural water birth and I ended up with a C section and following induced natural birth with complications), I am/my body is not good enough.*

Empowering thoughts that increase confidence are: *I've learnt to feel super-comfortable in my body despite the stretch marks and loose skin so much so that I wear a bikini and feel free in it, no matter what others think. I have two incredible boys that gifted me with a kind of love I only dreamed of before, they've made my life better in ways I couldn't ever imagine, my kids make my world beautiful and they make me want to live. No matter how they came, they're here in my life now.*

Considering my career and dreams, disempowering thoughts that decrease confidence are: *I tried different jobs but couldn't stick to any of them. I'm not a nutritionist, I don't have a medical degree, how can I write a book on weight loss.*

While empowering thoughts that increase confidence are: *I had the courage to change jobs and listen to myself and my passion and thanks to that I found what I really love doing and sticking to it it's now the easiest bit. I've lost 10kg and kept it off for 10 years, I have overcome food addictions and healed my distorted eating habits, I've been happy and free ever since and I've helped people do the same. I can definitely write a book where I share what has worked for us and I trust it will help others too.*

Do you see and feel the magnificent potency of this? Please give it a try. Put the book down right now and take a pen and paper. Come back to it -of course!, but for now, consciously change your thoughts and feelings to empower you, to trust yourself, to feel good within your skin. Your life will change, I promise.

You're stronger than you think you are, you're more powerful than you think you are, and you are way more loved than you think you are!

Chapter Summary

- It's quite possible for people lacking self-confidence to acquire this quality.

- Shift your focus and your perspective from disempowering to empowering reasoning.

Conclusion

Now you know how to lose weight naturally and permanently, while connecting with yourself and being more at home in your own skin. You also have a new relationship with food and your body. You are starting to nurture and feel a deep **connection** with yourself and experience a feeling of being at peace with what your body looks like. You're well on your way to being a new, healthy person who experiences more love, kindness, energy and progress on a daily basis, rather than fear, guilt, or overwhelm. Remember this is a mountain with no peak, and the better it gets the better it gets: your self-confidence will continue to increase the more you practice the principles and tools included in this book.

You're also more familiar at this point with distorted thinking patterns, those that lead to an unhealthy relationship with food, and even an eating disorder. Observing yourself and listening to your body will help you make the best choices for your mental and physical health, when you're eating alone, as well as with your family, and with friends.

Excessive dieting, restricting, and exercising are rarely sustainable ways to lose weight, and now you can leave those all in the rear-view mirror, along with your unhealthy body image and perception. Keeping in mind and applying the **80/20 rule** together with remembering that you **always** have a choice, will allow you to leave guilt behind and start enjoying every experience and every food more. Your journey inward is going to help you shine more and more brightly, and the wonderful part of this is that it will last for the rest of your life. Guilt, shame or pressure have no place in a healthy weight loss journey, and with the methods you've learnt in this book you can redefine your goals in a way that is without constraint and focuses on feelings and progress. The beauty of this work is that it evolves with you and its benefits are immediate *and* long lasting.

Start in the **Pole Position**, where you love yourself first, and your body then changes in response. Remember that you're navigating a course into new territory, so you'll need all of the tools available to you. Let this book be your map.

Always have your end goal at the forefront of your mind, where your relationship between your body and food is healed, and you've lost the amount of weight that you wanted to. That way, you'll be creating the feelings you want to experience, and you'll be happy with what you see in the mirror while being excited for what you are changing, instead of worrying about what the bathroom scales show. Acknowledge that you are worth it.

Decide and know that you won't give up. I have complete faith that you can do this because I have, and I have coached my clients to do the same.

Focus on your progress, what serves you and what supports you in your wellbeing and leave the rest behind. If you haven't succeeded in the past, you can always give yourself another chance. Be kind to yourself and at the same time take full responsibility for your behaviour and choices. Feel deeply worthy of love and belonging at all times because the truth is that you are!

Always have the **Bigger Picture** in mind, and remember your dreams. You have the capacity to achieve them. Go forward and make your dreams come true, always checking and processing and adjusting your feelings first. Listen to yourself to find out your true desires and associate them with feelings you would experience, for example feelings of being light and free, energetic, connected, in control, and inspiring to others.

Use the tools I have provided for you to write down your feelings and track your progress. It's essential to always have the Bigger Picture in mind to create a plan of action. That's how you'll be able to live your life full of confidence and gratitude, without limitations.

If you check in with yourself and you are not experiencing the feelings that you want to feel (attractive, sexy, lively, energetic, etc.), then use your tools of positive self-talk and positive affirmations to get there, and most importantly encourage yourself into loving yourself. Be your own biggest fan and best cheerleader. Leave the "shoulds" and "coulds" behind. You know what's funny? There's a new catch-phrase out in the world of mental and behavioural positivity that goes like, "Stop Should-ing Yourself." It is both funny and true. Don't think about what you should have done when you take a step backwards or make a mistake. Simply learn from it, accept it, and keep moving forward.

Always be kind and uplifting when you are talking to yourself, adopt a *'I'll figure it out and feel good throughout no matter what'* attitude which ultimately is the one that will most serve you. Don't forget about the power of experimenting with poses and saying heartening, cheerful, self-boosting affirmations to yourself in the mirror. It works and science has proven it. You *are* Superwoman or Superman. Believe that, and your body will believe it too. Always celebrate your efforts and reward yourself with positive reinforcement. People and animals are motivated by this, so when you set goals, reward yourself for each milestone you reach.

How we see ourselves subconsciously or unconsciously in our mind's eye really does matter, and that's been proven as well. Consciously change the way you walk to convey more confidence, and you will automatically *actually feel more confident*. Start laughing now, even if you have no reason for laughing, and you will automatically *actually feel happier* -

there's a whole branch of yoga called laughter yoga that is based on this concept. That's just the way it works. Internally remodel yourself! Remember to use your name in your "I" statements to yourself, so as to remove the anxiety and pressure and to replace it with a positive self-image statement.

Do and be your best in the here and now. Remember that there's no magic pill, you are the one with power, you are the one who can make this happen and who can allow support into your life to speed up the process and make it more pleasurable.

Forget the B.M.I. chart and all of your old ways of negative thinking and start fresh. I've said it before, and I'll say it again: *What we tell ourselves in our heads becomes our belief system, and our belief systems shape our behaviour.* So, always have your Bigger Picture **"Why"** at the forefront of your mind, and you'll feel guided and will be more empowered, you can't go wrong.

Then, remember your **F.F.F.s: Fear**, **Failure**, and **Forgiveness**. Remember that prevention is always better than a cure, and leave your past in the past. Don't make fear-based decisions. Instead, acknowledge and accept fear, and then call deep on your courage to *do what you're afraid of anyway.* Recall that failing and risking are necessary components of progress and success. Learn from your failures and keep progressing anyway. Remember Michael Jordan? The man failed thousands of times, but that didn't stop him. It helped him learn and become excellent at his trade.

Practice makes perfect, so don't be afraid to do the exercises and answer the prompts over and over, again and again. Your answers will evolve with you.

You are in control of your body, your behaviour, and what foods you put into your mouth, no one else is. Own it. Be the master of your life. You are not wrong or bad, no matter what has happened in your past. You are good and taking the right steps and decisions to be successful from now on. You have as many chances as you give yourself. Be raw and real and vulnerable with yourself, listen to what comes up and always be kind and loving like you were talking to your most beloved person.

Write down your feelings and take the time to think about and process them. Allow yourself the luxury of crying, freely. Remember that crying literally discharges pain from our bodies. It may not be the most comfortable thing to do, but it helps us heal and grow. Be kind to yourself and learn to love and nurture yourself, you are one hundred percent worth it.

Leave behind old ideas, traditions, and any beliefs that don't serve you. Believe that your desired outcomes are possible for you, and your thoughts, body, and behaviour will respond accordingly.

Bear in mind always that you, and you alone, can change your belief system for the better; it will take repetition and practice, but the reward is great. Don't buy into the negative things that you think about yourself. "This is just how I am," has no place in forging a new path through the wilderness and a new way of thinking and behaving. Acknowledge your insecurities, negative feelings and perceptions, and previous judgements about yourself, love on them, release them, and move forward.

Form a new, positive reality around and inside yourself by consciously changing your feelings and perceptions about what and how you are. Be the change you want to see. Learn to embody the confident, balanced, and energetic person you want to be-come.

Find your way, for example putting sticky notes with positive affirmations around your house, to remind yourself continuously of your new beliefs. Set time aside each day for positive self-talk and affirmations. Build them into your daily schedule. Remember that our sense of self-integrity as human beings depends on what we say to ourselves repeatedly. Keep up your global narrative in which you are at all times competent, moral, flexible, adaptive, and adequate.

We are not ever perfect - and that is perfectly okay. You are enough and always evolving. Black and white, inflexible thinking is useless and damaging. Blame and guilt are heavy and suffocating. Leave these things behind. You are doing a new thing. It is a new chapter in your book, and a new day has dawned.

You have stepped into your power, and you are more equipped now to successfully navigate and overcome negative things in your journey of confidence and growth. Being better to yourself is easy and fun, and you will become more and more enthusiastic about it.

Next, remember your **S.W.E.E.T. M.A.P.**, which is part of the scaffolding that you will be building your new, wonderful life and perceptions around. **Sleep**, **Water**, **Eating**, **Exit**, **Tracking**, **Mindfulness**, **Activity**, **Priority**. Quick fixes are not the answer, but a new way of living is. Implementing little changes on the daily will create the big changes you're after in your life. You now know that small changes can make an enormous difference in your life overall. You are motivated, you are strong, you are loved, and you deserve good things. We all do.

Every day, every moment is a good day and a good moment to commit to loving yourself, no matter what. Not giving up is the only way to get there. Make each day count and envision and so what would make your 8 years old and your 80 years old happy and proud.

You're already ahead of the game, far more than you imagine. What you desire is available to you, and you deserve it. You're so loved, way more than you think right now, and you're capable and strong beyond limits.

I am so very proud of you and it's been an honour sharing my precious methods for a happy and healthy life with you. You rock!

Sources

1. U.S. Department of Health and Human Services. "Calculate Your BMI." National Heart, Lung, and Blood Institute. https://www.nhlbi.nih.gov/health/educational/lose_wt/BMI/bmicalc.htm

2. Nordqvist, Christian. "Why BMI is Inaccurate." Medical News Today, August, 25, 2013. https://www.medicalnewstoday.com/articles/265215

3. Ahima, Rexford S., Lazar, Mitchell A. "The Health Risk of Obesity - Better Metrics Imperative." Science, Vol. 341, Issue 6148. August, 23, 2013. https://science.sciencemag.org/content/341/6148/856.summary

4. Jordan, Michael. "Twenty-three Michael Jordan Quotes That Will Immediately Boost Your Confidence." Inc. 5000, April 5, 2015. https://www.inc.com/benjamin-p-hardy/23-michael-jordan-quotes-that-will-immediately-boost-your-confidence.html

5. Kaur, Harmeet. "The Face of the Perseverance Landing was an Indian American Woman." CNN World, February, 19 ,2021. https://www.cnn.com/2021/02/19/world/swati-mohan-nasa-perseverance-landing-scn-trnd/index.html

6. Merriam-Webster. "The Merriam-Webster Dictionary." Merriam-Webster Inc., Encyclopaedia Brittanica, Inc.,

1828. https://www.merriam-webster.com/dictionary/gratitude

7. W. Bill. "Alcoholics Anonymous, The Big Book." Alcoholics Anonymous World Services., 1939. https://www.aa.org/

8. Ziv, Gal. "The Effects of Using Aversive Training Methods in Dogs--a Review." Elsevier, Journal of Veterinary Behavior. March, 18, 2016., https://www.sciencedirect.com/science/article/abs/pii/S1558787817300357

9. Cuddy, Amy. "Your Body Language May Shape Who You Are." TEDGlobal, Ideas Worth Spreading. May, 2012. https://www.ted.com/talks/amy_cuddy_your_body_language_may_shape_who_you_are?language=en

10. Mayo Foundation for Clinical Education and Research. "Anorexia Nervosa, Symptoms and Causes: Overview." Mayo Clinic. 1998-2021. https://www.mayoclinic.org/diseases-conditions/anorexia-nervosa/symptoms-causes/syc-20353591

11. National Eating Disorders Association. "Bulimia Nervosa: Diagnostic Criteria." NEDA. 2018. https://www.nationaleatingdisorders.org/learn/by-eating-disorder/bulimia

12. Mayo Foundation for Clinical Education and Research. "Body Dysmorphic Disorder: Symptoms and Causes Overview." Mayo Clinic. 1998-2021. https://www.mayoclinic.org/diseases-conditions/body-dysmorphic-disorder/symptoms-causes/syc-20353938

13. Govender, Serusha. "Is Crying Good for You?" WebMD, LLC. 2005-2021 https://www.webmd.com/balance/features/is-crying-good-for-you

14. Moore, Catherine. "Positive Daily Affirmations: Is There Science Behind It?" PositivePsychology.com. 3/1/2021. https://positivepsychology.com/daily-affirmations/

15. Popova, Maria. "Vincent Van Gogh on Fear, Taking Risks, and How Making Inspired Mistakes Moves Us Forward." Read It Later Inc. Pocket. Brain Pickings. Nov., 1, 2015. https://getpocket.com/explore/item/vincent-van-gogh-on-fear-taking-risks-and-how-making-inspired-mistakes-moves-us-forward?utm_source=pocket-newtab

16. Foley, Logan. Reviewed by Singh, Dr. Abhinav. "Why Do We Need Sleep?" The Sleep Foundation. September 11, 2020. https://www.sleepfoundation.org/how-sleep-works/why-do-we-need-sleep

17. Williamson AM, Feyer AM. Moderate sleep deprivation produces impairments in cognitive and motor performance equivalent to legally prescribed levels of alcohol intoxication. *Occup Environ Med.* 2000;57(10):649-55. https://www.cdc.gov/sleep/about_sleep/drowsy_driving.html

18. Arnedt JT, Wilde GJ, Munt PW, MacLean AW. How do prolonged wakefulness and alcohol compare in the decrements they produce on a simulated driving task? *Accid Anal Prev.* 2001;33(3):337-44.

https://www.cdc.gov/sleep/about_sleep/drowsy_driving.html

19. Dawson D, Reid K. Fatigue, alcohol and performance impairment. *Nature*. 1997;388(6639):235. https://www.cdc.gov/sleep/about_sleep/drowsy_driving.html

20. Mawer, Rudy, "17 Proven Tips to Sleep Better at night." Healthline. February 28, 2020. https://www.healthline.com/nutrition/17-tips-to-sleep-better

21. Leech, Joe. "7 Science Based Health Benefits of Drinking Enough Water." Healthline. June 30, 2020, https://www.healthline.com/nutrition/7-health-benefits-of-water#7.-Can-aid-weight-loss

22. Author Unknown. "The Benefits of Drinking Water for Your Skin." School of Medicine and Public Health, University of Wisconsin at Madison. https://www.uwhealth.org/madison-plastic-surgery/the-benefits-of-drinking-water-for-your-skin/26334

23. Laskowki, Dr. Edward R. "Sitting Risks: How Harmful is Too Much Sitting?" Mayo Clinic: Healthy Lifestyle: Adult Health. August 21, 2020. https://www.mayoclinic.org/healthy-lifestyle/adult-health/expert-answers/sitting/faq-20058005

24. Menga, Rich. Rich Menga Blog: Key to My Success. https://menga.net/3-liters-of-water-a-day

25. SugarStacker (Reddit name). "How much sugar is in soda pop?" Sugar Delirium Blog, Sugar Stacks, August 30, 2014. http://www.sugarstacks.com/blog/

26. Boyles, Salynn. "Soda Health Facts: Are Soft Drinks Really Bad for You? Sodas and Your Health: Risks Debated." WebMD. https://www.webmd.com/diet/features/sodas-and-your-health-risks-debated#1

27. Pase, Matthew. Himali, Jayandra. Beiser, Alexa. Aparicio, Hugo. Satizabal, Claudia. Vasan, Ramachandran. Seshadri, Sudha. Jaques, Paul F. "Sugar- and Artificially Sweetened Beverages and the Risks of Incident Stroke and Dementia." April 20, 2017. https://www.ahajournals.org/doi/10.1161/STROKEAHA.116.016027

28. Author Unknown. "Type 2 Diabetes: Symptoms and Causes. Mayo Clinic. https://www.mayoclinic.org/diseases-conditions/type-2-diabetes/symptoms-causes/syc-20351193

29. Eidem, Matthew. "Can Your Bowel Movement Be an Indicator of Digestive Health?" Digestive Health Blog. May 10, 2015. https://mattheweidem.com/can-your-bowel-movement-be-an-indicator-of-digestive-health/

30. Ellis, Esther. "Fiber." Academy of Nutrition and Dietetics: Eat Right. November 3, 2020. https://www.eatright.org/food/vitamins-and-supplements/nutrient-rich-foods/fiber

31. Quagliani, Diane. Felt-Gunderson, Patricia. "Closing America's Fiber Intake Gap." National Institutes of Health. July 7, 2016. https://www.ncbi.nlm.nih.gov/pmc/articles/PMC6124841/

32. Barone, Jeanine. "Can You Trust Calorie Counts on Food Labels?" Berkeley Health. September 20, 2016. https://www.berkeleywellness.com/healthy-eating/nutrition/article/can-you-trust-calorie-counts

33. Starecheski, Laura. "Why Saying is Believing--The Science of Self-Talk." NPR, WPSU Penn State. October 7, 2014. https://www.npr.org/sections/health-shots/2014/10/07/353292408/why-saying-is-believing-the-science-of-self-talk

34. Keiser, Anouk. Smeets, Monique. Dijkerman, Chris. Uzunbajakau, Siarhei. Van Elleburg, Annemarie. Postma, Albert. "Too Fat to Fit Through the Door." Plos One. plos.org. May 29, 2013 https://journals.plos.org/plosone/article?id=10.1371/journal.pone.0064602

35. Kross, Ethan. Bruehlman-Senecal, Emma. Moser, Jason. Park, Jiyoung. Burson, Aleah. Dougherty, Adrienne. Shablack, Holly. Bremner, Ryan. "Self-Talk as a Regulatory Mechanism: How You Do It Matters." American Psychological Association. Journal of Personality and Social Psychology, 2014, Vol. 6, No. 2, 304-324. http://selfcontrol.psych.lsa.umich.edu/wp-content/uploads/2014/01/KrossJ_Pers_Soc_Psychol2014Self-talk_as_a_regulatory_mechanism_How_you_do_it_matters.pdf

36. Gaudiano, Brandon A. "Cognitive Behavioral Therapies: Achievements and Challenges." U.S. National Library of Medicine. National Institutes of Health. February 11,

2008.
https://www.ncbi.nlm.nih.gov/pmc/articles/PMC367329
8/

37. Lee, I-Min. Shiroma, Eric J. Kamada, Masamitsu.
"Association of Step Volume and Intensity With All-
Cause Mortality In Older Women." JAMA, Internal
Medicine. 2019; 179 (8): 1105-1112.
https://jamanetwork.com/journals/jamainternalmedicine/f
ullarticle/2734709

38. Morris, Martha Clare. Wang, Yamin. Barnes, Lisa L.
Bennett, David A. Dawson-Hughes, Bess. Booth, Sarah L.
"Nutrients and Bioactives in Green Leafy Vegetables and
Cognitive Decline." Neurology. January 16, 2018.
https://www.ncbi.nlm.nih.gov/pmc/articles/PMC577216
4/

39. Shea, M Kyla. Kritchevsky, Stephen B. Loeser, Richard F.
Booth, Sarah L. "Vitamin K Status and Mobility
Limitation and Disability in Older Adults: The Health,
Aging, and Body Composition Study." The Journals of
Gerontology: Series a. The Gerontological Society of
America. May 6, 2019.
https://academic.oup.com/biomedgerontology/advance-
article-
abstract/doi/10.1093/gerona/glz108/5485918?redirectedF
rom=fulltext

40. Author Unknown. "Blame and Rigid Thinking: They're
Undermining Your Mental Health." Exploring Your
Mind. February 21, 2018.

https://exploringyourmind.com/blame-rigid-thinking-mental-health/

41. Kang, Sonia K. Galinsky, Adam D. Kray, Laura J. "Power Affects Performance When the Pressure is On: Evidence for Low-Power Threat and High-Power Lift." Sage Journals. April 17, 2015. https://journals.sagepub.com/doi/abs/10.1177/01461672 15577365

42. Cascio, Christopher N. Brook O'Donnell, Matthew. Tinney, Francis J. Lieberman, Matthew D. Taylor, Shelley E. Strecher, Victor J. Falk, Emily B. "Self-affirmation Activates Brain Systems Associated with Self-Related Processing and Reward and is Reinforced by Future Orientation." Oxford Academic, Social and Affective Cognitive Neuroscience. Volume 11, Issue 4, Pages 621-629. April 2016. https://academic.oup.com/scan/article/11/4/621/2375054

43. https://www.youtube.com/watch?v=hE2lna5Wxuo

44. OxfordLanguages. Oxford Languages and Google. Definition of "mindfulness." Oxford University Press. 2021. https://languages.oup.com/google-dictionary-en/

45. Saint-Maurice, Pedro. Troiano, Richard P. Matthews, Charles E. Kraus, William E. "Moderate-to-Vigorous Physical Activity and All-Cause Mortality: Do Bouts Matter?" Journal of the American Heart Association. Vol. 7. No. 6. March 22, 2018. https://www.ahajournals.org/doi/full/10.1161/JAHA.117. 007678

46. Helmer, Jodi. "Dancing for Exercise: Ballroom, Hip Hop, Latin, and More." WebMD. JumpStart. August 2, 2020. https://www.webmd.com/fitness-exercise/a-z/dance-for-exercise

47. Lawler, Moira. "What is Self-Care and Why is it Critical for Your Health?" Everyday Health. April 5, 2020. https://www.everydayhealth.com/self-care/

48. Author Unknown. "What Do We Mean by Self-Care?" World Health Organization. WHO 2021. https://www.who.int/reproductivehealth/self-care-interventions/definitions/en/

49. Trollope, Anthony. "An Autobiography" Project Gutenberg. Chapter Twenty, 'The Way We Live Now.' Release date, 2012. http://www.gutenberg.org/ebooks/5978

www.ingramcontent.com/pod-product-compliance
Lightning Source LLC
Chambersburg PA
CBHW032104280326
41933CB00009B/753